ATHLETIC TRAINING
CASE SCENARIOS

**Domain-Based Situations
and Solutions**

ATHLETIC TRAINING
CASE SCENARIOS
Domain-Based Situations and Solutions

EDITED BY

KEITH M. GORSE, EDD, LAT, ATC
Assistant Professor/Clinical Coordinator
Department of Athletic Training
Duquesne University
Pittsburgh, Pennsylvania

FRANCIS FELD, MS, MED, CRNA, LAT, ATC, NRP
Staff CRNA, UPMC Passavant Hospital
Prehospital RN, Ross West View and Penn State EMS
Supervisor, Allegheny County Hazmat Medical Team
Supervisory Nurse Specialist, PA-1 DMAT
Pittsburgh, Pennsylvania

ROBERT O. BLANC, MS, LAT, ATC, EMT-P
Athletic Trainer—Football, University of Pittsburgh
Adjunct Clinical Faculty, School of Health and Rehabilitation Sciences
University of Pittsburgh
Pittsburgh, Pennsylvania

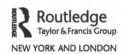

Routledge
Taylor & Francis Group

NEW YORK AND LONDON

First published in 2016 by SLACK Incorporated

Published 2024 by Routledge
605 Third Avenue, New York, NY 10158

and by Routledge
4 Park Square, Milton Park, Abingdon, Oxon OX14 4RN

Routledge is an imprint of the Taylor & Francis Group, an informa business

Library of Congress Cataloging-in-Publication Data

Gorse, Keith M., author.
  Athletic training case scenarios : domain-based situations and solutions / Keith M. Gorse, Francis Feld, Robert O. Blanc.
     p. ; cm.
  Includes bibliographical references and index.
  ISBN 978-1-61711-981-1 (alk. paper)
  I. Feld, Francis, - , author. II. Blanc, Robert O., - , author. III. Title.
  [DNLM: 1. Athletic Injuries--diagnosis--Case Reports. 2. Athletic Injuries--diagnosis--Examination Questions. 3. Athletic Injuries--therapy--Case Reports. 4. Athletic Injuries--therapy--Examination Questions. 5. Sports--Case Reports. 6. Sports--Examination Questions. 7. Sports Medicine--methods--Case Reports. 8. Sports Medicine--methods--Examination Questions. QT 18.2]
  RD97
  617.1'027--dc23
                          2015015163

ISBN: 9781617119811 (pbk)
ISBN: 9781003522676 (ebk)

DOI: 10.4324/9781003522676

DEDICATION

To all of the educators and clinicians who have worked hard, through their own experiences, to prepare athletic trainers in the past, present, and future.

CONTENTS

Dedication .... *v*
Acknowledgments .... *ix*
About the Editors .... *xi*
Contributing Authors ....*xv*
Preface .... *xix*

Section I   **Scenarios and Resolutions**.. **1**

Chapter 1   Domain I: Injury/Illness Prevention and Wellness Protection 3

Chapter 2   Domain II: Clinical Evaluation and Diagnosis 31

Chapter 3   Domain III: Immediate and Emergency Care 89

Chapter 4   Domain IV: Treatment and Rehabilitation 141

Chapter 5   Domain V: Organizational and Professional Health and
              Well-Being 171

Section II   **Appendices**... **225**

Appendix A   Glossary of Sports Medicine Terms 227

Appendix B   Athletic Training Terminology 243

Appendix C   Suggested Readings in Athletic Training 245

Appendix D   National Athletic Trainers' Association Position, Official, Consensus,
              and Support Statements.. 247

Bibliography *251*
Financial Disclosures..*253*
Index..*257*

ACKNOWLEDGMENTS

During the year that *Athletic Training Case Scenarios: Domain-Based Situations and Solutions* has been in production, many persons have assisted us. The staff at SLACK Incorporated was supportive and patient during the entire process of developing this textbook. In particular, we thank Brien Cummings, who provided the continuing support that gave us the initial okay to proceed and make it happen.

We thank the National Athletic Trainers' Association (NATA) and all of its members for allowing us to put together a comprehensive set of scenarios and situations that cover each of the 5 educational domains in athletic training.

Most importantly, we thank all of our contributors to this textbook. They openly shared their real-life athletic training scenarios; this shaped this textbook into the book we want to present to all certified and student athletic trainers for review and discussion.

Keith M. Gorse thanks the faculty and staff in the Rangos School at Duquesne University for allowing him the time to work on this textbook. Keith also thanks his family (Betsy, Erin, and Tyler) for the support they have given through the years. Last but not least, Keith thanks Hempfield Area High School, Carnegie Mellon University, Shady Side Academy, Middle Road Athletic Association, and Fox Chapel Baseball Association, where many of his real-life scenarios occurred over the past 33 years.

Francis Feld thanks Christine and Zoe for their love, support, and understanding every time a new project came up over the years. He also acknowledges the many athletic trainers and paramedics who shared rainy and snowy nights working with him to care for patients as best they could. The relationships built on the field or in the back of an ambulance are forged in steel, last forever, and are priceless.

Robert O. Blanc thanks his wife, Peggy, and all of his family members for their support and patience with the lifestyle that is athletic training. Also, to the physicians, faculty, staff, and students at the University of Pittsburgh over the past 27 years who have given so much of themselves to teach, learn, and advance this great profession—he is proud to have stood by you, and he looks forward to a great future.

ABOUT THE EDITORS

Keith M. Gorse, EdD, LAT, ATC is an assistant professor at the Rangos School of Health Sciences at Duquesne University in Pittsburgh, PA and also serves as the Clinical Coordinator for the Undergraduate Athletic Training Program.

Dr. Gorse received his bachelor of arts degree in Secondary Education and Athletic Training from the University of Pittsburgh (1983), and his master of education degree also from the University of Pittsburgh (1988). He spent 2 years working at Hempfield Area High School in Greensburg, PA and 15 years at Carnegie Mellon University in Pittsburgh. While working at Duquesne University, Dr. Gorse received his doctoral degree in Education (2010).

Dr. Gorse has been teaching in the Athletic Training Program since 2001. His areas of instruction have included sophomore-level introduction to athletic training, athletic injury evaluation, emergency care, applied science, and administrative issues in health care. In that time, Dr. Gorse has also been Clinical Coordinator for all sophomore-, junior-, and senior-level students. The Athletic Training Program uses over 30 different clinical education sites (on and off campus) and 65 different clinical education preceptors.

Dr. Gorse's research interests include commotio cordis, youth sports injuries, and emergency care issues. He has published 7 peer-reviewed manuscripts and contributed to over 14 professional presentations in his areas of research expertise. Additionally, Dr. Gorse has co-authored one academic text book in athletic training and is currently co-authoring another athletic training text book that will be published in 2015.

Dr. Gorse is a member of the National Athletic Trainers' Association (NATA), the Eastern Athletic Trainers Association, the Pennsylvania Athletic Trainers' Society (PATS), the American Heart Association (AHA), and the American Red Cross. Professionally, Dr. Gorse spent 5 years (2006-2010) serving as a member of the programming committee for the NATA Annual Meeting and Clinical Symposium, and 6 years (1998-2004) as the District II Rep for the NATA College/University Committee. He was chair of the NATA Age Specific Task Force for 3 years (2003-2005). He routinely serves as a moderator and/or program reviewer for the NATA Annual Meeting. He currently is a member of the NATA Sponsor Review Committee and acts as the Alleghany County Rep to PATS. Dr. Gorse has been an instructor in CPR, AED, and First Aid for both the AHA and American Red Cross for the past 25 years. He teaches and certifies students, coaches, and teachers both on campus and off campus at local schools and youth sport associations.

Dr. Gorse is a licensed athletic trainer through the Pennsylvania State Board of Medicine. He has over 30 years of clinical experience, working at both the high school and college levels. At Hempfield High School, Dr. Gorse served as their first full time athletic trainer. During his time at Carnegie Mellon University, Dr. Gorse was the head athletic trainer for over 17 men's and women's varsity sports and also taught in the Physical Education department. Currently, Dr. Gorse does some outside clinical work with Shady Side Academy Middle and High School in Pittsburgh, working with various varsity sports, including the baseball and ice hockey programs. Dr. Gorse has also been a coach/manager for various youth baseball programs in the Shaler and Fox Chapel school districts, also in Pittsburgh, for the past 14 years.

Francis Feld, MS, MEd, CRNA, LAT, ATC, NRP is a Certified Registered Nurse Anesthetist at UPMC Passavant Hospital in Pittsburgh, PA, where he specializes in thoracic anesthesia. Prior to working at Passavant, he spent 16 years at UPMC Mercy Hospital, which is a Level One Trauma and Burn Center where he specialized in cardiac and trauma anesthesia. Mr. Feld is active in the prehospital arena as a paramedic for Ross West View EMS in Pittsburgh and Penn State University EMS in University Park, PA where he works home football games. A portion of his duties with Ross West View EMS is covering 2 local high school football teams as a paramedic. He is Medical Group Supervisor for the Allegheny County Hazardous Materials Medical Response Team and is a supervisory nurse specialist for the Federal PA-1 Disaster Medical Assistance Team. Mr. Feld was deployed for Hurricanes Gustav, Lee, and Sandy; the Haiti Earthquake; and several National Security events. He has completed terrorism training at the Center for Domestic Preparedness in Anniston, AL where the training included work with live nerve and biological agents.

Prior to entering the EMS and nursing fields, Mr. Feld worked as a certified athletic trainer at Center High School in Beaver County (now Central Valley), the University of Pittsburgh, and the Pittsburgh Steelers. He has worked the summer games of the Special Olympics for 18 years at Penn State as a volunteer athletic trainer and as a paramedic. He is the Co-Editor of the textbooks *Emergency Care in Athletic Training* and *Athletic Training Case Scenarios: Domain-Based Situations and Solutions*. Mr. Feld has been a member of the National Athletic Trainers Association (NATA) since 1973 and a certified member since 1976. He serves as a core member of the writing group that has prepared the NATA's position statement on the appropriate prehospital care of spinal injuries. He has lectured at the local, regional, state, and national levels on emergency care, cardiac care, spine and orthopedic injuries, emergency planning, and disaster response.

Mr. Feld holds a BA in history and a MEd in sports administration from the University of Pittsburgh, a BSN from Duquesne University in Pittsburgh, and a MS in nursing anesthesia from LaRoche College in Pittsburgh. He is currently pursuing a Doctor of Nursing Practice degree at Carlow University in Pittsburgh and is Regional Faculty for the American Heart Association in ACLS, PALS, and BLS.

Robert O. Blanc, MS, LAT, ATC, EMT-P enters his 28th year as head football athletic trainer and clinical instructor at the University of Pittsburgh in PA. With his exceptional sports medicine knowledge and experience, Blanc is a tremendous resource for the entire University of Pittsburgh athletic department.

Blanc was named the 2013 NCAA Division I Head Athletic Trainer of the Year by the National Athletic Trainers' Association (NATA). He was selected for this prestigious award by the NATA College and University Athletic Trainers' Committee, which annually recognizes individuals for exceptional performance as a head athletic trainer in each of the 5 collegiate divisions (Divisions I, II, and III; NAIA; and junior college).

In addition to his responsibilities with the Pittsburgh Panthers' football program, Blanc has a lead role with the University of Pittsburgh Performance Team, a unique blending of the university's numerous resources that focuses on the development and welfare of the total student-athlete. He also helps coordinate sports coverage, budget, inventory, drug testing, and counseling.

Blanc is an adjunct clinical instructor for the University of Pittsburgh's NATA-approved undergraduate athletic training curriculum. He has co-authored 2 textbooks, *Emergency Care in Athletic Training* and *Athletic Training Case Scenarios: Domain-Based Situations and Solutions*, with 3 graduates of the University of Pittsburgh athletic training program.

Blanc graduated from Slippery Rock University in PA in 1982 and earned his master's in athletic training in 1984 from Ohio University in Athens. He was also a certified paramedic and was involved in an emergency medical service for 17 years in nearby Bethel Park.

A native of Pittsburgh, Blanc served as head athletic trainer at Duquesne University in Pittsburgh for 2 years before joining the Panthers' staff. Blanc began his athletic training career as the head athletic trainer at New Lexington (Ohio) High School in 1983. One year later, he began working for the Pittsburgh Steelers on a part-time basis, serving at the training camp and at all home games.

Contributing Authors

Jon Almquist, ATC
Vienna, Virginia

Adam Annaccone, MEd, ATC, AT, PES, CES
Phoenix, Arizona

Lynn Bott, MS, ATC, LAT
Lawrence, Kansas

Rick Burr, MS, LAT, CSCS
Natick, Massachusetts

Rex Call, LAT, ATC
Greencastle, Indiana

Eric Cardwell, MS, LAT, ATC
Pittsburgh, Pennsylvania

Douglas J. Casa, PhD, ATC
Storrs, Connecticut

Robert J. Casmus, MS, LAT, ATC
Salisbury, North Carolina

Craig Castor, MS, LAT, ATC
Venetia, Pennsylvania

Jim Cerullo, PhD, ATC
University Heights, Ohio

Kevin M. Conley, PhD, ATC
Pittsburgh, Pennsylvania

Larry Cooper, MS, LAT, ATC
Harrison City, Pennsylvania

Ron Courson, ATC, PT, NREMT-I, CSCS
Athens, Georgia

Jennifer Doherty-Restrepo, PhD, ATC, LAT
Miami, Florida

A. J. Duffy III, MS, ATC, PT
Norwood, Pennsylvania

Tim Dunlavey, MS, LAT, ATC
Pittsburgh, Pennsylvania

Scott Frowen, MS, LAT, CSCS
West View, Pennsylvania

Timothy K. Giel, MS, LAT, ATC
Gibsonia, Pennsylvania

Al Green, MEd, LAT, ATC, EMT
Lakeland, Florida

Michael Hanley, MS, LAT, ATC
Greenville, North Carolina

Kelley Henderson, MEd, LAT, ATC
Estero, Florida

Timothy J. Henry, PhD, ATC
Brockport, New York

Valerie W. Herzog, EdD, LAT, ATC
Ogden, Utah

Adam M. Hindes, MS, LAT/C, CSCS
Oakmont, Pennsylvania

Peter Houdek, LAT, ATC
Quakertown, Pennsylvania

Peggy A. Houglum, PhD, ATC, PT
Gibsonia, Pennsylvania

Chuck Kimmel, LAT, ATC
Boone, North Carolina

Mary K. Kirkland, MS, ATC, LAT
Kennedy Space Center, Florida

Catherine S. Lenhardt, LAT, ATC
Chapel Hill, North Carolina

Sarah Manspeaker, PhD, ATC
Forth Worth, Texas

Christopher Marrone, MPT, LAT, ATC
McKees Rocks, Pennsylvania

Randy McGuire, MS, ATC
Georgetown, Kentucky

Jennifer McKenzie, MSEd, LAT, ATC
Pittsburgh, Pennsylvania

Linda P. Meyer, EdD, LAT, ATC
Central City, Pennsylvania

Sayers John Miller, PhD, PT, LAT, ATC
State College, Pennsylvania

Mary Mundrane-Zweiacher, PT, ATC, CHT
Middleton, Delaware

Kathleen Nachazel, LAT, ATC
Pittsburgh, Pennsylvania

Gregory Nordlund, ATC
Wheaton, Illinois

John Panos, MEd, LAT, ATC
Pittsburgh, Pennsylvania

David H. Perrin, PhD, ATC, FNATA
Greensboro, North Carolina

Ben Potenziano, MEd, LAT, ATC
Pittsburgh, Pennsylvania

Marirose Radelet, MS, ATC, PT (Retired)
Pittsburgh, Pennsylvania

Matthew Radelet, PA-C, AT (Retired)
Tucson, Arizona

Jeramiah Randall, PT, LAT, ATC
Pittsburgh, Pennsylvania

Richard Ray, EdD, ATC
Holland, Michigan

Joan Reed, ATC
Clarkston, Georgia

Christopher Rose, MS, LAT, ATC
Pittsburgh, Pennsylvania

Gaetano Sanchioli, MS, LAT, ATC, PES
Pittsburgh, Pennsylvania

Bonnie J. Siple, EdD, LAT, ATC
Cranberry Township, Pennsylvania

Rebecca L. Stearns, PhD, ATC
Storrs, Connecticut

Charles Thompson, MS, ATC
Lawrenceville, New Jersey

Todd Tomczyk, MS, LAT, ATC
Pittsburgh, Pennsylvania

Paula S. Turocy, EdD, LAT, ATC
Bethel Park, Pennsylvania

Giampietro L. Vairo, PhD, ATC
University Park, Pennsylvania

Brian Vesci, MA, ATC
Brighton, Massachusetts

Michael Vittorino, MS, LAT, ATC
Moon Township, Pennsylvania

Mary C. Wisniewski, ATC
Chicago, Illinois

PREFACE

Athletic Training Case Scenarios: Domain-Based Situations and Solutions is intended to assist readers with critical thinking and knowledgeable resolutions to true-life scenarios that may occur in each of the 5 domains of athletic training education. Many textbooks give 1 or 2 scenarios or case study–type questions at the end of each chapter; however, it is the intent of this textbook to provide readers with many true-life scenarios that have occurred and have been shared by certified athletic trainers currently working with industrial, high schools, colleges, professional teams, and sports medicine clinics. It is our intent to include scenarios/situations and resolutions listed for each of the domains listed in the National Athletic Trainers' Association (NATA) Board of Certification.

Section I contains the scenarios, discussion questions, and resolutions to the scenarios that cover each of the educational domains in athletic training. In Section II, the appendices list medical and athletic training terminology as well as the different NATA position, official, consensus, and support statements.

After a few years of building on this idea, it is pleasing to see our concept take shape and to see this textbook become a reality. It is our hope that *Athletic Training Case Scenarios: Domain-Based Situations and Solutions* will be an asset to student and certified athletic trainers and that it will serve as a critical-thinking guide to many scenarios and resolutions in athletic training.

Keith M. Gorse, EdD, LAT, ATC
Francis Feld, MS, MEd, CRNA, LAT, ATC, NRP
Robert O. Blanc, MS, LAT, ATC, EMT-P

I

SCENARIOS AND
RESOLUTIONS

1

Domain I
Injury/Illness Prevention and Wellness Protection

SCENARIO 1: COMPLIANCE ISSUES WITH A LACROSSE GOALIE

Two weeks into the college season, the goalie on the women's lacrosse team presented to the athletic trainer with multiple, severe contusions on both of her lower legs. The goalie indicated that she suffered several direct blows to both shins when stopping the ball in goal. Shin guards are available but are not required for goalies in collegiate women's lacrosse. The contusions were painful, with significant ecchymosis and visible edema causing decreased strength in the tibialis anterior muscle of both shins. She also presented with an antalgic gait and foot slap when walking. Appropriate treatment soon returned her strength and function. Upon resolution of the signs and symptoms of the contusions, the athletic trainer was prepared to return the goalie to play on the condition that she wear shin guards or another fabricated form of protection on both shins during practices and games. The goalie refused to wear the shin guards.

Discussion Questions

1. What options does the athletic trainer have at this point?

2. Who can assist the athletic trainer in resolving this situation?

3. What condition(s) could result from further contusions to this soft tissue?

Gorse KM, Feld F, Blanc RO, eds.
Athletic Training Case Scenarios:
Domain-Based Situations and Solutions (pp 3-30).
© 2016 Taylor & Francis Group.

Resolution

The athletic trainer educated the goalie about the risks of further contusions to the shins without the protection of shin guards or other padding, but the goalie continued to refuse to wear shin protection. The athletic trainer addressed her concerns and criteria for return to play to the coach and indicated she would not clear the goalie unless she wore shin protection. The coach supported the athletic trainer's decision that the goalie needed to wear shin protection. The goalie still refused to wear shin protection, so the coach did not let her play. The goalie sat out for 1 week while continuing treatments and not practicing or playing in games before agreeing to the athletic trainer's criteria for return to play. The goalie experienced no further contusions and played the remainder of the season without injury. Unfortunately, while away from campus over the summer, the goalie played lacrosse and did not wear any form of shin protection. As a result of multiple contusions over the summer, the athlete experienced bilateral anterior compartment syndrome and a stress fracture to the right tibia, which resulted in her inability to play during the next college season.

Additional Resolution

The athletic trainer would have urged the coach to require the goalie to continue to wear her shin guards during the summer when playing lacrosse in goal.

Notes:_____

_____

_____

_____

_____

_____

Scenario 2: Asthma in Collegiate Women's Soccer

A certified athletic trainer was working with a college women's soccer team during a training session. At the end of the session, the coach decided to have the team work on fitness, and timed sprinting intervals began. The athletic trainer noticed an athlete who appeared to be struggling to recover more than the others between sprints. Eventually, the athlete removed herself from the drill and bent over to try to catch her breath. The athletic trainer approached her and asked if she was okay. The athlete nodded her head to indicate "yes." The athletic trainer suggested that she try to stand upright and walk a bit to get her breathing under control. Then, the athletic trainer asked the athlete if she had asthma. The athlete nodded her head "yes." The athletic trainer then asked the athlete if she used her inhaler prior to the training session. The athlete shook her head "no" and pointed to the sideline where there were 20 or more identical backpacks. The athletic trainer eventually located the athlete's backpack and retrieved the inhaler. After using her rescue inhaler, the athlete slowly recovered and her breathing returned to normal.

Discussion Questions

1. What could the athletic trainer have done differently to take care of this athlete in a more expeditious manner?

2. When would you call emergency medical services (EMS) for an asthma attack?

3. What criteria should be used to return this athlete to participation?

Resolution

The athlete took 2 puffs of her inhaler and resumed normal breathing in 10 to 15 minutes. The athletic trainer asked the soccer player why she did not use her inhaler prior to soccer training, and the athlete responded, "No one else has to use an inhaler." The athletic trainer found that her peripheral capillary oxygen saturation percentage was within normal limits, and peak flow measurements were within normal limits for the athlete's age, sex, and height. The athletic trainer then educated the athlete on why she needed to use the inhaler and reviewed proper use of an inhaler. The soccer player was cleared to return to full participation by the team physician and was instructed to report any further signs and symptoms to the athletic trainer.

*Notes:*_____

_____

_____

_____

_____

_____

SCENARIO 3: GUNSHOTS AT YOUTH FOOTBALL PRACTICE

An athletic trainer's athletes were practicing on 2 different fields about 3 city blocks apart on the same street. The athletic trainer was required to monitor both fields during practices. One evening, as the athletic trainer was leaving one field for the other, 3 gunshots rang out nearby. The young players on the field where the trainer was currently positioned appeared unaffected, although the coaches and parents had become wary. The athletic trainer proceeded to the other field, where she found disarray but no injuries. Some of the players had run off. Coaches, parents, and players reported that a car had slowly circled the field, then drove down to the street below the field and started shooting at someone.

Discussion Questions

1. Is practice cancelled? On both fields?

2. Whose responsibility is it to find the players who ran?

3. How would you set up a policy to deal with extreme and dangerous issues such as this?

Resolution

The athletic trainer's Emergency Action Plan and Standard Operating Procedures now has a section on gunshots that reads, "In the event of gunshots on or near the field, all coaches will yell loudly, 'Get down! Get down! Get down!' and then enforce the directive. This directive will apply to everyone on the field."

Editor's Note

Active shooter scenarios are all too common in society today, and every organization must have a written plan for such events. The plan must be formulated in conjunction with local law enforcement and public safety officials. These events can occur in any location, not just a school, so it is important for community athletic organizations to also have a plan. In this case, it is crucial that all athletes are accounted for and that they are safely in the care of a responsible adult.

*Notes:*_____

_____

_____

_____

_____

_____

SCENARIO 4: COACH CHALLENGING AUTHORITY FOR PLAYER SAFETY

The home team athletic trainer was working a big high school rivalry soccer game prior to the playoffs. The athletic trainer was in charge of both teams because the visiting team did not bring an athletic trainer. One of the opposing team's players sustained a head injury after colliding with another player while going up for a head ball. When directed to by the official, the athletic trainer ran out on the field to perform an initial assessment and to determine how to get the athlete removed from the field. The player was guided off on his own; however, the athletic trainer noticed signs of a possible concussion while doing the initial assessment. A full secondary evaluation was performed on the sidelines to confirm the possibility of a concussion, and the athlete was told that he should not go back into the game because of the injury. The athletic trainer spoke to the opposing team's head coach to let him know that the athlete should not return to the game because of the possibility of having a concussion. The coach of the team did not listen to the athletic trainer and put the player back into the game.

Discussion Questions

1. Who has jurisdiction in this case when a visiting team does not bring an athletic trainer?

2. How could the communication in this situation have been better between the home team athletic trainer and visiting team? What should the home team athletic trainer have done before the game to keep this issue from occurring?

3. If the home team athletic trainer is providing medical coverage for the visiting team, should the schools have a written contract in place delineating the responsibilities of the athletic trainer and who will make return-to-play decisions?

Resolution

After an appropriate stoppage in the game, which luckily was just a few minutes with no physical contact by the injured player, the athletic trainer signaled the official to remove the player from the game. The athletic trainer went to the coach, relayed his dismay, and told the coach that the player could be injured worse if he had another head-to-head contact with a player during that game. The coach then decided to keep the player out for the rest of the game.

Notes:_____

_____

_____

_____

_____

_____

SCENARIO 5: DEVELOPMENT OF A COMPREHENSIVE WELLNESS PROGRAM

With the increased demands on students in regard to classroom/homework, practice, and work/internships, it was determined by the athletic director and sports medicine staff that more emphasis needed to be placed on the overall health and well-being of student athletes. The athletic population within the school had numerous students over the past few years who had displayed abnormal behavior due to the inability to cope with these demands and an inert need to improve or maintain a certain performance/image. This behavior spawned unhealthy habits in the form of eating disorders and increased substance abuse, as well as increased signs of stress, anxiety, and depression. Not only was this affecting the students' classwork and their ability to cope with the rigors of school, it was also affecting their ability to perform at their optimal level on the playing field. The issue was brought up to the entire Sports Medicine/Performance Team, and it was determined that we needed some form of education in place as well as a method to determine which athletes may be at greatest risk. The Performance Team included the athletic training staff, team physician, athletic director, sports nutritionist, health services (university medical director, university nutritionist, and wellness coordinator), and counseling services. The team members were asked to provide what they considered risk tendencies for their area of expertise and a method of determining who may display or be at risk of developing these tendencies. They were also asked if they were willing to participate in brief educational sessions in their areas of expertise.

Discussion Questions

1. What type of risk tendencies could you potentially see in student athletes, and why would this be the concern of the athletic training staff?

2. What methods could you use to determine if your student athletes were at risk of potentially harmful tendencies, and how would you address these issues?

3. In what ways could this program evolve to better address the needs of the student athlete population?

Resolution

After many meetings with the performance team, a comprehensive wellness form was developed for student athletes to complete at the beginning of every school year. This form includes questions regarding supplement and drug use, depression, nutrition, and alcohol use. The sections are scored based on national testing data, and athletes who are considered at risk are referred to the team physician and/or members of the program (nutritionist, wellness coordinator, and counselors). Athletes are also subject to testing (blood work, electrocardiogram, drug testing, etc) as determined by the team physician and/or other members of the team. Athletes' compliance in the program is mandatory, and those determined at risk must follow through with the plan determined by the team physician or they risk restrictions to participation. In addition to the wellness questionnaire, all athletes must also participate in the yearly educational sessions provided. These sessions are brief 30- to 60-minute discussions given to the teams regarding alcohol and substance abuse, nutrition, and stress management, as well as how to contact health and counseling services if needed.

Additional Resolution

The wellness program is constantly evolving. We review the program yearly and meet with all members of the team to determine how the year went and if any changes need to be made. We also consult with the student athlete advisory council to get their ideas on improvements to the program in regard to the educational sessions, what they feel is most beneficial, and what may be lacking.

Notes:_____

_____

_____

_____

_____

_____

SCENARIO 6: OSTEOPENIA IN A FEMALE ATHLETE

A female track athlete and cheerleader was treated for shin pain early in her freshman track season. Further evaluation with unsuccessful rehabilitation and localizing point tenderness indicated referral. Following full work-up, she was diagnosed with bilateral stress fractures and discontinued from play to continue rehabilitation.

Her sophomore track season started well, but her pain returned within 1 week. Rehabilitation was again initiated, and her activity level was modified to give some relief. When no improvement was noted, she was referred again. X-rays and bone scans were negative. Blood tests and dual energy x-ray absorptiometry scanning to determine diet and/or bone mineral deficiencies were negative. She was prescribed several vitamin and mineral supplements for her diet. She was unable to complete her sophomore season.

She was able to rest and continue cheerleading the next fall without pain. She started light workouts in the winter with a gradual build-up to running just prior to the track season. She is running with some pain but not at the level she had felt the prior 2 years.

Discussion Questions

1. How would you structure an offseason workout regimen to benefit this athlete?

2. What modalities, pre- and postexercise, would most benefit this athlete?

3. Which vitamins and minerals would most benefit this athlete?

Resolution

This athlete continues to do preventative exercises for flexibility and strength of her hips, legs, ankles, and feet. The athletic trainer has had her gait assessed in running and walking, and has worked with the sprint coach to make corrections to her running pattern. She is wearing flats specific to her problem for practice.

Her training consists of a stepwise build-up to meet day (25%, 50%, 75%, meet, off-day, 25%, etc). She does a pool workout of shallow and deep water running 1 day per week. The athletic trainer had completed a lower body assessment of tender points and has begun positional release therapy to address any dysfunction that may contribute to her pain.

Notes:
_____

_____

_____

_____

_____

_____

SCENARIO 7: WRESTLING A NEW OPPONENT

During wrestling season, we had 2 teams—the varsity and junior varsity—go to away tournaments. When they came back on Monday, we had multiple wrestlers with suspicious lesions on the right sides of their faces and foreheads. Closer examination revealed 2 very different skin conditions. Some looked like herpes gladiatorum, and others appeared to be impetigo. Either way, we had to investigate in case it was herpes gladiatorum to stop its spread. What complicated things was the number of teams at each tournament and determining who had direct or indirect contact. Using a regional athletic trainer database, I sent emails to all 45 athletic trainers and/or athletic directors from the teams that were registered at the tournament.

Almost immediately, I received phone calls from each school. They had many questions about which wrestler, what they should do, what the next steps were, etc. Although we were not the first school to go through this situation, there was no policy in place on how to handle an outbreak of either condition. All that was available were recommendations on how to treat the skin condition on the athlete. To complicate matters, we had a match in 3 days.

Because this was considered a communicable disease outbreak, I reported the situation to the local county health agency, the local and state athletic association directors, the state department of health, the State Sports Medicine Advisory Committee Chair, and local physicians. We convened an emergency meeting for the Sports Medicine Advisory Committee along with physicians from the state and county departments of health. All physicians involved stated that the 2 conditions were difficult to distinguish in the early stages and that it was imperative that treatment begin immediately to control the skin conditions.

Discussion Questions

1. Should the entire team be quarantined? Is 2 weeks enough time for the lesions to clear up?

2. Is it necessary to contact each school that had wrestlers in attendance at the tournaments?

3. Do you feel that this situation was handled correctly? Why or why not?

Resolution

It was decided that the wrestling team should be quarantined for a minimum of 14 days. They could still condition, shadow wrestle, and lift; however, no skin-to-skin contact with any other wrestler was allowed. It was also suggested that the wrestlers who were formally diagnosed with herpes gladiatorum be put on a prophylaxis regimen or to treat active disease with acyclovir 400 mg 3 times daily until the wrestling season was over.

Our wrestlers were given prescriptions for acyclovir for the remainder of the season, and all wrestlers were able to complete the season with no occurrence of the herpes gladiatorum.

*Notes:*_____

_____

_____

_____

_____

_____

SCENARIO 8: NOT ALL ATHLETIC SHOES ARE CREATED EQUAL

During the winter season a few years ago, I noticed that there was an abnormally large number of ankle sprains among our basketball players—young men and women at all levels. I saw this through the thorough injury statistics that were collected. This information motivated me to investigate equipment, shoes, practice drills, previous injury rates, and previous injuries to the affected student athletes. Unfortunately, none of this turned up any significant information or injury trends. Next, I called some neighboring secondary school athletic trainers and asked them a series of questions. This collaboration was invaluable.

I found out that some other athletic trainers had noticed more ankle sprains than usual and could not figure out the cause. Then, I noticed that all of the schools that I contacted were also wearing the same brand of shoe. It was a team shoe and was relatively new as far as the style and bells and whistles that it was promoting.

Discussion Questions

1. Should you collaborate with other athletic trainers? If yes, how would collaboration with other athletic trainers benefit you?

2. Are there other ways that the statistics could help you? List any that you can see.

3. Does this type of information help make your job more secure? Why or why not?

Resolution

At this time, I went to the National Athletic Trainers' Association list-serve and posed a few questions to the members. The response was overwhelming—members across the country were seeing the same injury trends associated with this team shoe. Armed with this information, I was able to go to our basketball coaches and athletic director and change the type of shoe that we purchased to prevent future injuries.

The following year, we saw a return to normal ankle injury rates, and I found that the shoe was discontinued due to defects during the manufacturing process.

Notes:_____

_____

_____

_____

_____

_____

SCENARIO 9: FOOTBALL HUDDLE COLLAPSE

Two certified athletic trainers were covering a collegiate football game away from home. At the end of the game, an athlete on the home team collapsed during the team huddle. Once the athletic trainers arrived on the scene, they noticed that the athlete was unconscious and breathing heavily. At that time, the ambulance and team doctors for the home team had already left the field to go home. The visiting team's athletic trainers came over to assist with the injured athlete. An athletic trainer cut off his jersey and shoulder pads. An automated external defibrillator was retrieved in case it was needed. The local EMS was alerted. The EMS stated that the ambulance that was at the game was on another call and they would have to send another ambulance crew, which would take about 10 to 15 minutes. After a few minutes, the athlete stopped breathing multiple times for a period of about 5 seconds each. The athlete had a history of asthma. Once the EMS arrived on the scene, they took over and intubated the athlete. It was determined that the athlete needed to be airlifted off the field to get appropriate medical treatment. The athlete was loaded into a helicopter and taken to the appropriate hospital.

After the game, other athletes on the team told the athletic trainers that the athlete was complaining of concussion-like symptoms during the first half of the game but hid it from the athletic trainers. During the last drive of the game, the athlete was kicked in the head during a play. No one on the team told the athletic trainers about the symptoms or incidents during the game.

Discussion Questions

1. What condition(s) would you, as an athletic trainer, be worried about in this situation?

2. Was it appropriate for the team doctor and EMS to leave the field before all athletes were off the field?

3. What could you do as an athletic trainer to help prevent this situation from occurring in the future in any sport? What information is important to document immediately after the incident?

Resolution

The athlete in this scenario was cleared to try and return to football about 1.5 years after the incident, but the athlete never returned to full competition again. The athlete struggled with cognitive functions after the incident for the remainder of his collegiate career. The athlete continuously had symptoms while working out.

After the incident, the athletic trainer reviewed the concussion policy at the school and Emergency Action Plan to make sure all proper steps were taken. Revisions of both plans were taken into consideration. Both schools were in contact after the games to get documentation together to make sure all odds and ends were together.

*Notes:*_____

_____

_____

_____

_____

SCENARIO 10: ATHLETE WITH POTENTIAL EATING DISORDER

During the fall preseason, an athletic trainer contacted the head volleyball coach about a student athlete who had returned to college with various overuse injuries in her lower legs. The athletic trainer also mentioned that, after reviewing medical paperwork for the volleyball team, he noticed a significant weight loss in the student athlete from the previous spring. The head coach revealed that he had been approached by a few of his players that the student athlete has been missing team meals and had been reclusive. The teammates were concerned that the student athlete might have an eating disorder.

Discussion Questions

1. How would you approach the student athlete regarding the potential weight loss?

2. What resources would you use to help the student athlete with a potential eating disorder?

3. Are there any regulations regarding the health status and who you can talk with about the student athlete?

Resolution

The athletic trainer expressed a concern for the student athlete because her current body mass index was at 15.8 kg/m^2, which was considered at risk and was down from 18.2 kg/m^2 in the spring. The athletic trainer met with the student athlete to discuss the number of injuries she had during preseason and that her coach had expressed concern about her. During the discussion, the athletic trainer explained to the student athlete the importance of nutrition in preventing injuries as well as during the healing phases of an injury. The athletic trainer asked the student athlete if she had been making sure she was eating between practices. The student athlete said it had been difficult because she had been tired and trying to catch up on her sleep between practices and that she was not hungry. The athletic trainer mentioned that, in reviewing her medical history, her weight was down from the spring. The athletic trainer explained that body mass index is a tool that is used to measure a person's weight based upon their height, and that she was low. The athletic trainer sympathized with the student athlete that it is difficult to eat properly at times and suggested that she make an appointment with the college nutritionist to help her make better choices about foods that she can eat between and after practices. Based on Family Educational Rights and Privacy Act and Health Insurance Portability and Accountability Act regulations, the athletic trainer asked the student athlete if it was okay to contact the nutritionist and provided only the information they talked about in the meeting. The student athlete agreed. The athletic trainer called the college nutritionist to give her a heads up that the student athlete would be calling her and expressed the concerns he had about the student athlete. The nutritionist and the athletic trainer have been actively working together to identify athletes of concern with regard to eating issues.

*Notes:*_____

_____

_____

_____

_____

_____

SCENARIO 11: MEDICATION ISSUE FOR ICE HOCKEY INJURY

A high school ice hockey player was told by his parents to take medication for the swelling he was experiencing in his shoulder after an injury that occurred during a varsity hockey game on Saturday afternoon. The player was told by his mother and father to take 2 Tylenol (acetaminophen) tablets 4 times per day until he saw the athletic trainer on Monday afternoon. The athlete went to the athletic training facility after classes that following Monday and explained to the athletic trainer that he felt no better and that the swelling had gotten worse over the previous 36 hours. The athlete explained to the athletic trainer that he had been taking Tylenol like his parents had instructed him to do after the game. The athlete did not do any other type of treatment after the game until now (ie, ice and compression). The athletic trainer explained to the athlete that Tylenol is not an anti-inflammatory drug and that he should have been icing the shoulder and using a compression wrap to help alleviate the swelling and inflammation.

Discussion Questions

1. What type of over-the-counter medications and dosages should the athlete be taking to help alleviate swelling and inflammation issues to the injured shoulder?

2. What precautions should be pointed out when explaining to athletes the problems with using anti-inflammatory drugs without proper education regarding the usage of such medications?

3. What are the adverse effects that athletic trainers should be looking for in an athlete taking anti-inflammatory drugs?

Resolution

The athletic trainer had to explain to the student athlete that Tylenol is not an anti-inflammatory and that taking it would not reduce swelling in his injured shoulder.

There should be a specific protocol in the Athletic Training Facility–Standard Operating Procedures that provides information to student athletes and parents on the proper use of over-the-counter medications. Over-the-counter medications should not be given or taken by an injured athlete without proper education and direction of use by a physician or athletic trainer.

*Notes:*_____

_____

_____

_____

_____

_____

SCENARIO 12: WRESTLING ADMINISTRATION AND MEDICAL CONDITIONS

An athletic trainer assessed a wrestler on a Monday with what resembled a herpes cluster on the right temporal area of his head. Approximately 1 hour later, 2 more wrestlers were sent to the athletic training room with the same signs and symptoms.

The athletic trainer determined that it was not a coincidence that 3 members from the same varsity team had what was perceived to be herpes gladiatorum. They were all evaluated by the team physician and their private pediatricians for the diagnoses. Once diagnosed, the questions of how and why this virus occurred on a team that had not competed in over 8 days arose. The facility mat surface was disinfected before and after practice with bleach-soaked towels to step on prior to entrance to the wrestling room.

Discussion Questions

1. How was the virus contracted?

2. Who should be notified (by law) of this incidence?

3. What should be done with the wrestling facility after the diagnosis has been made?

Resolution

The team had open mat, and 3 wrestlers who had been carriers infected the team. Unfortunately, the alumni were not forthcoming initially.

The medical staff held a question-and-answer period with the athletes, parents, and coaching staff. Treatment and pretreatment options were discussed. By Pennsylvania law, the parents of the high school were notified of the outbreak and the solution to the situation.

The wrestling team was not permitted to participate in practice or competition for 4 days. The athletic facility was closed and cleaned. No activity occurred within the self-standing building or field house for the 4 days during the cleaning process.

Notes:_____

_____

_____

_____

_____

_____

SCENARIO 13: DISPENSING MEDICATION FOR ILLNESS

An athletic trainer in the athletic department of a large university was working in the treatment center over the summer when one of the coaches came in saying he was not feeling well and asked to speak with the athletic trainer who covered his team. The athletic trainer took the coach over to an examination table and began speaking to him. He got a stethoscope and auscultated the coach's chest for several minutes. He then went into the team physician's examination room and returned with what another trainer recognized as a prescription pill bottle. He gave this to the coach. The trainer who had witnessed the transaction knew that the team physician was on vacation; the trainer later asked a colleague about the dispensing of medication, and he said that he gave the coach antibiotics after the team physician instructed him to do so over the phone.

Discussion Questions

1. Do antibiotics need to be kept in locked cabinets? What are the medical–legal implications for athletic trainers having access to prescription medications?

2. Should the dispensing athletic trainer have been asked about the situation or do you think it would have been more properly handled by addressing the team physician or head athletic trainer first?

3. What other options are there for the coach to receive appropriate medical care without going to the athletic trainer or team physician?

Resolution

Once the team physician returned from vacation, the head athletic trainer held a staff meeting to resolve the issue of whether athletic trainers should dispense prescription medications with a verbal order from the physician. All agreed that the legal language could be interpreted in slightly different ways. It was therefore decided that, in the future, athletic trainers would not dispense prescription medications, even with consent and direction of the team physician. This policy, although perhaps slightly inconvenient at times, allowed for legal protection of the athletic trainers, the team physician, and the university.

Notes:_____

_____

_____

_____

_____

_____

SCENARIO 14: PREVENTING HEAT ILLNESS ON AN ABNORMALLY WARM DAY

It was an abnormally hot day in mid-March, and an athletic trainer was working a lacrosse game. The temperature had averaged 60°F to 62°F the past few weeks. The field had been too wet to practice outside most days. During game time, the athletic trainer read that that day's temperature would be pushing 80°F to 82°F.

The athletic trainer provided both teams with water and ice as was done for every game. One of the lacrosse athletes mentioned to the athletic trainer that the goalie was not feeling well before the game. When the athletic trainer approached the goalie and made conversation, he seemed fine and said he was feeling good and ready for the game.

The athletic trainer kept an eye out on the goalie throughout the day. During the second half of the game, the athletic trainer suddenly noticed that he was hunched over in front of his goal. He did not lose consciousness, but he stated that he just wanted to rest for a minute. Upon further questioning, he said that he felt dizzy and his vision was a bit blurry. The athletic trainer told the athlete to come out of the game and take his goalie equipment and helmet off. He also had the athlete get out of the hot environment and into the athletic training facility for additional medical assessment.

Discussion Questions

1. What condition was the lacrosse goalie suffering from during the game?

2. What are the signs and symptoms for heat-related illness and initial care for an athlete suffering from heat-related illness?

3. What can the athletic trainer do to prevent conditions like this from occurring in the hot weather environment?

Resolution

The athletic trainer did a complete medical assessment to determine the lacrosse goalie's condition, and it was determined that the athlete was suffering from heat syncope. Once in the athletic training facility, the athlete's core body temperature was taken orally, and it was a bit higher than 99°F. The goalie was still sweating profusely, so the athletic trainer asked the goalie to sit in the air conditioned room with just a shirt and shorts on. The athlete was also given an electrolyte drink to sip on while he rested. After about 35 minutes in the facility, the athlete was feeling better, and his body temperature had gone back down to normal (98.6°F). The athlete was instructed not to play for the rest of the game and to keep hydrated when he got back to his dorm room. The athlete was released once all signs and symptoms of the heat syncope had gone away. No further medical assistance was needed, and the athlete was told to come back to the athletic training facility the next day for a quick re-evaluation.

Notes:_____

_____

_____

_____

_____

_____

Domain II
Clinical Evaluation and Diagnosis

SCENARIO 1: HEAD INJURY IN NONCONTACT FOOTBALL DRILLS

In October 2012, Princeton University Football was entering the fourth week of their season. They were 2-2 and 1-0 in the Ivy League, coming off a commanding win vs a nonconference opponent and heading into their second conference game. As was typical, there was the injury check-in and treatments the following day, followed by meetings and a brief, light workout. Monday was the players' day off, with medical care being the only expectation.

Tuesday's practice was a full-pad practice, which was the usual schedule. Even with full pads, the schedule called for a very minimal amount of full contact drills. The normal schedule for a Tuesday practice was followed. Each position or group spent the majority of the start of practice working on warm-ups and individual techniques. The second phase of practice had started, which consisted of special teams work. There is no live contact involved with any special team drills, with shields being used primarily. The athletic training staff was engaged in functional rehabilitation with a group of injured players.

During the course of the special team drills, one of the defensive backs came to the medical staff with one of his teammates and told us that he thought something was not right with the teammate. He returned to practice, and the medical staff began their examination.

Gorse KM, Feld F, Blanc RO, eds.
Athletic Training Case Scenarios:
Domain-Based Situations and Solutions (pp 31-88).
© 2016 Taylor & Francis Group.

The injured athlete was initially alert and wakeful but was complaining of a headache focused on the frontal part of the head. His headache quickly worsened, and he failed to answer questions related to orientation. He also had no recollection of the previous game, including the opponent, win or loss, etc, and he also became very emotional, which was out of character for him. He was typically animated, funny, and self-deprecating.

During the initial evaluation on the field, he was originally oriented. *The Sport Concussion Assessment Tool, Third Edition* (SCAT3) was started, and he was 0/5 on modified Maddocks Questions; immediate word recall was 15/15, but delayed recall was 0/5. His pupils were equal and reactive to light, his cranial nerves were intact, his cervical spine was nontender, and upper and lower extremity strengths were normal.

The decision was made to have him transported by ambulance to the local hospital, which is approximately 1 mile from campus. He was brought into the athletic training room while waiting for the ambulance, at which time he began vomiting. The team physician made the decision that he should be taken to the trauma center, which was approximately 10 miles from campus. The normal protocol for the ambulance was to transport to the closer hospital, but, after a firm conversation with the team physician, they transported him to the trauma center.

Within 30 minutes of being transported, he had a bolt in his skull to monitor the pressure in his head, as well as a shunt. It was determined through a cerebral angiogram that he had an arteriovenous malformation within the left ventricle distal to the anterior cerebral artery. Surgery was performed to resect the malformation.

Discussion Questions

1. How does an athletic trainer differentiate between a concussion and a more serious head injury, such as was presented, or a subdural or epidural hematoma?

2. What arrangements/agreements should the athletic trainer have with the local emergency medical services (EMS) service in regard to transportation issues?

3. What was the significance of the teammate's awareness of the need to bring his teammate to the attention of the medical staff?

Resolution

This athlete has made a full recovery. He has been cleared by the neurosurgeon for full participation in football activities. Repeat cerebral angiogram was performed 1 year postoperatively, and everything was normal. He returned to school at the start of the Fall 2013 academic year and has performed very well in the classroom.

He was allowed to begin physical training at this time. There was a slow and gradual progression of cardiovascular and strength training exercises. At the start of the Spring 2014 semester, he resumed football drill work and participated in the full offseason football program. Later that semester, he participated in 12 days (maximum allowable by Ivy League rules) of football practice without incident or issues.

Prior to the start of these activities, his parents were involved in intensive discussions regarding his return. He had no reservations regarding his return and exhibited no signs of hesitation while playing. Because he played cornerback, he was not typically involved with a high number of collisions, but he was to be called upon to make high speed tackles when the 2014 season started.

Additional Resolution

In hindsight, it was obvious that the decision to force the transportation of this athlete to the trauma center may have saved his life and helped to assure a positive outcome.

Notes:_____

_____

_____

_____

_____

_____

Scenario 2: Femoral Shaft Stress Fracture

A 21-year-old female lacrosse attacker reported left groin and hip pain but denied any acute trauma. She was evaluated late in the fall season and had pain over the adductor and lateral pubic tubercle. After conservative measures failed, an injection at the adductor origin was performed. Three months later, during the middle of her senior season, she again reported pain in the hip area. Further questioning revealed that pain now extended into the left thigh and knee area. The examination revealed full knee and hip active range of motion (ROM) and stable joints but pain with internal rotation of the hip. She reported no neurologic symptoms. Complicating her presentation was a history of a surgically repaired distal femur fracture in high school with hardware subsequently removed. The athlete was initially treated with rest, 400 mg of ibuprofen 4 times daily, cryotherapy, and electrical muscle stimulation, but she was subsequently referred to the team physician for further evaluation. Initial x-rays showed a cortical irregularity in the proximal femur. A bone scan confirmed a femoral shaft stress fracture. The athlete insisted that she be allowed to play as it was her senior year and last season of eligibility. Her coach wanted her to keep playing because she was one of the few experienced and talented players on this relatively new sport just added to the athletic program.

Discussion Questions

1. Who has the final say on whether an athlete should be allowed to play following an injury diagnosis?

2. What is the appropriate immediate care for an athlete with a diagnosed stress fracture?

3. What information should the certified athletic trainer relay to a coach regarding stress fracture injury prevention and care?

Resolution

The athlete was withheld from athletic activity and instructed not to bear weight for 3 weeks. She was permitted to perform upper body strength training and swimming for cardiovascular conditioning. Following 3 weeks of nonweightbearing, the athlete was advanced to partial weightbearing with crutches for 2 weeks, encouraged to continue her aquatic therapy, and began riding a stationary bike. Follow-up x-rays at 6 weeks revealed a resolved femoral stress fracture. The athlete was permitted to begin a return-to-play regimen over the next 2 weeks. She then returned to full activity and participated in the latter part of the competitive lacrosse season without further incident.

*Notes:*_____

_____

_____

_____

_____

_____

SCENARIO 3: MALLET THUMB INJURY

A 22-year-old male football player at the center position reported immediate pain and loss of mobility of the left thumb after striking an opponent's shoulder pad breast-plate during a collegiate football game. The initial sideline examination revealed a flex-ion deformity at the thumb interphalangeal (IP) joint and inability to extend the distal phalanx actively as well as against applied resistance. The athlete had no pain to palpa-tion of the proximal phalanx but had mild pain dorsally over the IP joint. The patient had no tenderness at the metacarpophalangeal joint, and stress testing of the collateral ligaments was negative. The team physician performed a confirmatory sideline evalu-ation and the injury was diagnosed as a mallet thumb injury. The athlete wanted to continue playing and the coaching staff encouraged him to return to the game as soon as he could.

Discussion Questions

1. Who has the final say on whether an athlete should be allowed to play following an injury diagnosis?

2. What is the appropriate immediate care for an athlete with a mallet finger injury?

3. What is the proper splinting protocol for an athlete with a mallet finger injury?

Resolution

The athlete was placed into a commercial polyethylene splint designed to treat mallet fingers, and closed-cell foam padding was applied for additional protection. The athlete was allowed to return to play and he completed the contest without further incident. Following the game, the athlete kept the thumb IP joint splinted in full extension. The next day, x-rays were taken and revealed no evidence of fracture. The athlete was evaluated by the team orthopedist and the involved extremity was placed into a short-arm thumb spica cast. The athlete wore the cast with closed-cell padding for football-related activities for the next 10 days. The cast was then removed and the athlete was placed back into the commercial polyethylene splint with closed-cell padding for an additional 18 days. After this time, the athlete wore padded gloves over the commercial splint and participated in all football activities for the next 12 days. When not participating in sports activities, the athlete was instructed to continuously wear the commercial splint with the IP joint in full extension. At the conclusion of the season, the athlete was re-evaluated by the team physician and orthopedist. The player had no extension lag, had full active IP joint extension and flexion, and was able to flex and extend the distal phalanx of the thumb against applied resistance. The athlete was instructed to wear the commercial splint at night for an additional 2 weeks; otherwise, he was permitted full activity with no restrictions.

Editor's Note

All thumb injuries must be taken seriously because a poor outcome can lead to a lifelong disability. Only the ability to reason and opposable thumbs separate humans from other primates.

*Notes:*_____

_____

_____

_____

_____

_____

SCENARIO 4: HYPERTHYROIDISM ISSUE IN FOOTBALL PLAYER

A 22-year-old male transfer football player presented to the athletic training room for his annual preparticipation examination with reports of palpitations, hot flashes, eye bulging, and nervousness for the past 3 months. He had seen a physician at home who prescribed eye drops. He denied visual changes or depression. He denied a family history of thyroid disorders. Physical examination showed an anxious, muscular male in no acute distress. Blood pressure was 140/70, pulse was 88 beats per minute, and body weight was 210 lb (down from 223 lb). A Snellen eye chart examination revealed 20/25 right eye vision and 20/20 left eye vision. There was mild left greater than right exophthalmos. He had no appreciable goiter, mucous membranes were moist, and he had no heart murmurs. The athlete was entering his final year of eligibility and was highly regarded as a prospect to play football professionally upon graduation. The athlete wanted to be cleared to play immediately, and the coaching staff was looking forward to his participation.

Discussion Questions

1. What key signs and symptoms made a referral to a medical specialist such as an ophthalmologist and an endocrinologist necessary?

2. Why is hydration so important per physical activity of this athlete in question?

3. What information should the certified athletic trainer relay to a coach regarding hyperthyroidism treatment and care?

Resolution

The athlete was referred to an ophthalmologist and thyroid tests were ordered. His thyroid-stimulating hormone was less than 0.02 uIU/mL (range, 0.46 to 4.68 uIU/mL), triiodothyronine was greater than 20.0 pg/mL (range, 2.3 to 4.2 pg/mL), and thyroxine was greater than 6.99 ng/mL (range, 0.64 to 1.92 ng/mL). He was then referred to an endocrinologist; however, prior to the consultation, he developed a goiter and heat intolerance and lost an additional 7 lb. He was then withheld from football activity except for weightlifting and conditioning drills as tolerated, with an emphasis on proper hydration. The medical staff also found out that his mother, grandmother, and 2 aunts had a history of hyperthyroidism. His thyrotropin receptor antibody was 26.9 u/L (range, 0.0 to 1.0). He was diagnosed with moderately severe Graves' disease and was started on methimazole and adjunctive therapies, including cholestyramine, metoprolol, eye drops, and vitamin D. After 3 weeks of therapy, he developed neutropenia, with a neutrophil count of 0.57. The athlete was then referred to an ear, nose, and throat (ENT) specialist, who recommended thyroidectomy. Following his uneventful surgery, he was weaned off of his medications and permitted to begin cardiovascular conditioning exercises. He was cleared to begin running 5 days postoperatively. He was permitted to begin noncontact football agility drills 10 days postoperatively. Two weeks postoperatively, he was allowed to return to all football-related activities and was permitted limited playing time in a varsity contest 17 days post-thyroidectomy. He returned to full, unrestricted football activity 8 weeks after initial presentation in the athletic training room.

Notes:_____

_____

_____

_____

_____

_____

SCENARIO 5: ISOLATED FIRST RIB FRACTURE

A 20-year-old male football player was struck on the right shoulder during a kickoff return drill during a collegiate football practice. The athlete reported immediate pain and pain with forward flexion. The initial examination revealed anterior shoulder pain and inability to forward flex and abduct the shoulder with applied resistance. The athlete had no pain to palpation over the acromioclavicular joint but had moderate pain along the distal scapula. He had no tenderness along the cervical spine and moderate pain along the superior trapezius. Full cervical spine ROM was noted. There was no clavicle pain or deformity. No glenohumeral instability was noted and glenoid labrum tests were deferred. No pain occurred with respiration and no neurovascular symptoms were noted. The athlete was treated with ice, placed in an arm sling, and told to report to the athletic training room the next morning for further evaluation and care. Upon reporting for follow-up the next day, the athlete stated that his pain now radiated more intensely to the posterior-superior scapular region. He was then referred to the team physician for evaluation and x-rays, which revealed a transverse fracture to the first rib. The team physician determined that this injury needed to be managed conservatively, as these types of injuries can have concomitant injuries to surrounding neurovascular structures if not properly managed. This particular injury would require at least 3 to 4 weeks of care and rehabilitation prior to any return to full-contact football activity. The involved athlete did not want to lose 1 year of eligibility by returning for the latter part of the football season. He wanted to pursue a medical redshirt and sit out the remaining portion of the football season. The coaching staff viewed this injury as a generic rib fracture and wanted the athlete protectively padded to continue playing for the remainder of the season.

Discussion Questions

1. Who has the final say on whether an athlete should be allowed to play following an injury diagnosis?

2. Why is radiating pain a concerning symptom during injury evaluation and diagnoses?

3. What is the appropriate immediate care and rehabilitation for an athlete with a diagnosed rib fracture?

Resolution

The athlete remained in the arm sling and withheld from football activity but was permitted to ride a stationary bike for exercise. The use of thermal modalities began 72 hours post-trauma. At 10 days, the athlete was free of pain with glenohumeral ROM and began rotator cuff exercises with the elbow adducted using elastic tubing. Glenohumeral joint distraction was aggravating and was, therefore, avoided. The athlete could begin forward and lateral dumbbell raises from 45 to 90 degrees as no pain was elicited along with biceps and triceps strengthening and seated rows using elastic tubing. At 2 weeks, repeat x-rays revealed a continued fracture line with no evidence of bony union, and the athlete was point tender over the superior trapezius muscle. He also had pain with resisted cervical motion. There was no neurovascular compromise to the upper extremity. When not participating in therapy, the athlete was instructed to wear the arm sling and refrain from overhead activity. Repeat x-rays at 6 weeks showed moderate bony calcification beginning to occur at the fracture site. At 10 weeks, x-rays showed the fracture site with full bony union. Because of the time loss from football activity, the athlete successfully applied for a medical hardship waiver. The athlete is currently asymptomatic and has returned to all athletic and daily living activities.

*Notes:*_____
_____
_____
_____
_____
_____

SCENARIO 6: EVALUATION AND RECOGNITION OF BREATHING DYSFUNCTION

During football preseason, a high school athlete was having difficulty breathing during the conditioning sprints. He presented with shortness of breath and tightness in the chest causing dizziness. No wheezing was noted on evaluation. At the time, the athletic trainer pulled the athlete from practice and referred him to a cardiologist for evaluation. The cardiac evaluation came back as normal and the athlete was released back to play. As the season went on and conditioning decreased, the athlete did not present with symptoms again. The athlete then went on to play basketball and had a reoccurrence of the signs and symptoms, but they subsided with rest. He was able to compete throughout the season. The following football preseason, the athlete presented with the same symptoms. Upon questioning, the athlete stated that this had been happening throughout the summer and he had been to 2 doctors to be evaluated for asthma, which came back as negative. He was never given a diagnosis. With more questioning by the athletic trainer, the athlete stated that there was a feeling of tightness at the throat and an inability to pass air to the lungs, and the athlete appeared to be gulping for air. The athletic trainer continued with the history and found that it only happened with heavy exertion in all environments. With the history and signs and symptoms, the athletic trainer referred him to an ENT for possible vocal cord dysfunction.

Discussion Questions

1. What are signs and symptoms of respiratory conditions?

2. What are the differential diagnoses?

3. What other appropriate referrals could have been made?

Resolution

After evaluation by an ENT, paradoxical vocal cord dysfunction was diagnosed and the athlete was given breathing exercises and medication to control the issue. The athlete returned to play and has been able to control the dysfunction.

Notes:_____

_____

_____

_____

_____

_____

SCENARIO 7: ANKLE SPRAIN IN A PROFESSIONAL BALLET DANCER

An athletic trainer determined that a principal ballet dancer sustained an ankle injury while being set down from a partner lift on stage during a professional ballet performance. The dancer was sitting in the wings offstage with her dance slippers on and did not want to remove them as she hoped to immediately return to the performance if she was physically able.

The ballet dancer was complaining of minimal medial ankle pain, minimal decreased active ROM, and no apparent strength deficits. There was no obvious swelling, discoloration, or deformity. Anterior glide, bump, and compression tests were all negative. The dancer got up and was able to walk and perform small jumps with minimal pain.

Due to severe time constraints, the athletic trainer was not able to perform a comprehensive physical evaluation but determined that the dancer had suffered a medial ankle sprain and could return to dance provided modifications in the performance could occur.

Discussion Questions

1. Do you think the dancer should be removed from the performance and a comprehensive evaluation be performed? Why or why not?

2. What components of an injury evaluation are crucial to determine if the dancer is capable of returning to the performance?

3. What, if anything, should be done to help stabilize the dancer's ankle to return to the performance?

Resolution

The athletic trainer performed a comprehensive evaluation of the dancer's injury after the performance and determined that the findings were the same. The dancer had sustained a mild medial ankle sprain. The athletic trainer recommended ice, compression, and elevation. She was offered crutches for the evening but declined. The following day, the dancer was re-evaluated prior to the performance and was found to have full, active, pain-free ROM; 5/5 strength in all directions; and negative bump, compression, and anterior glide tests. She returned to the performance without limitations.

*Notes:*_____

_____

_____

_____

_____

_____

SCENARIO 8: FRACTURED FEMUR

An athlete was injured during a kickoff in football. He was on the receiving team and was blocking when he was struck by an opposing player and went down. The patient was unable to bear weight and was in pain. On and off the field, the patient complained of knee pain. On the sideline, the knee was evaluated, and no obvious ligamentous laxity or other internal derangements of the knee were noted. There was no obvious deformity or classic fractured femur signs and symptoms. The player did not report thigh or hip pain. The player was assisted to the sideline, sat on the bench, and was re-evaluated throughout the game. The knee was placed in a knee immobilizer and was iced during the game. His signs and symptoms were monitored during the game. Because an ambulance was on-site, the player was transported by ambulance to the hospital for x-rays and an additional examination. Upon radiological examination, a mid-shaft fracture was noted.

Discussion Questions

1. What dilemma does it cause an athletic trainer when the athlete's perception of the injury is different than the actual injury?

2. When treating an acute injury, what steps can or should an athletic trainer take to insure that they are taking in consideration other possible injuries or secondary conditions?

3. Why is referred pain to the knee common with hip and femur injuries? Explain.

Resolution

Following the discovery of the femur fracture, the player was admitted and underwent a surgically implanted rod the next day. Following 1 year of rehabilitation, the player resumed all football activities for the next football season.

*Notes:*_____

_____

_____

_____

_____

_____

SCENARIO 9: SOFTBALL PITCH TO FACE

An athletic trainer was covering a home softball game. During the game, an athlete on the home team was attempting a slap hit; the pitch was wild and struck her in the face. The athlete was not wearing a protective facemask on her helmet at the time of injury. She fell to the ground crying and holding her face. The athletic trainer was summoned on the field by the umpire.

At the time of arrival, the athletic trainer noticed severe inflammation of the right cheek. There was deformity of the zygomatic bone in the right cheek. The athlete was also displaying epistaxis from her right nostril. There was no bruising at the time of arrival. There was pain with movements of the eye looking both down and out, and there was pain with movement of the jaw.

After the athletic trainer calmed the patient down, the athletic trainer had the athlete slowly sit up. Once the athlete sat up, she stated that she was dizzy and that there was a pain in the back of her neck. At that time, the athletic trainer had the athlete lay back down and started inline stabilization of the neck. Once the athlete laid back down, the pain in her neck and the dizziness disappeared. At that time, the emergency action plan (EAP) was activated and EMS was called. Once EMS arrived on the scene, the athlete was spine boarded and taken to the hospital for further treatment.

Discussion Questions

1. What injuries would you as the athletic trainer be concerned about in this scenario?

2. Should you as an athletic trainer ever go with an athlete to the hospital? How would you decide if you had to go to a hospital with an athlete?

3. What are the potential complications of placing an athlete with a nose bleed supine? What equipment should be readily available?

Resolution

After the game, the athletic trainer was notified that the athlete had a fracture of her right zygomatic bone and required cosmetic surgery to fix the problem. She also sustained a mild concussion with the injury. There was no injury to the cervical spine.

After 3 weeks of recovery and a new facemask, the athlete was back on the field playing with the team again.

*Notes:*_____

_____

_____

_____

_____

_____

SCENARIO 10: COLLEGE BASEBALL PITCHER

An athletic trainer was evaluating a right-hand–dominant college baseball pitcher in the training room following his removal from a game due to right shoulder pain. The athlete reported that he felt immediate pain in his shoulder following one pitch. He was unable to continue pitching in the game due to this discomfort as he could not throw without significant pain. He reported no previous right shoulder or elbow injuries. He rated his pain level at 2/10. Immediately after he threw his last pitch, he rated his pain as 6/10. He displayed no decrease in velocity or accuracy during the game.

He presented with the following clinical evaluation.

Observation

- No effusion/edema, discoloration, or deformities present.

Postural Evaluation

- The following things were revealed upon ocular observation:
  - Forward head
  - Bilaterally rounded shoulders
  - Bilaterally internally rotated humerus
  - Increased thoracic kyphosis
  - Right scapula (inferior angle) was lower compared to the left scapula

Active Range of Motion

- All shoulder planes were within normal limits.
- Pain was reported above 90 degrees of flexion.
- Pain was reported above 90 degrees of abduction.

Strength

- Full can test: 4/5 with pain reported
- External rotation at 0 degrees of shoulder abduction: 4/5 with pain reported
- Internal rotation at 0 degrees of shoulder abduction: 5/5 with no pain reported
- External rotation at 90 degrees of shoulder abduction: 4/5 with pain reported
- Internal rotation at 90 degrees of shoulder abduction: 4/5 with pain reported

Special Tests

- Speed's test: (–) for pain
- Dynamic Speed's test: (–) for pain
- Yergason's test: (–) for pain
- Apprehension test: (–) for pain/apprehension
- O'Brien's test: (+) for pain and weakness
- Anterior Slide test: (+) for pain
- Biceps Load test: (+) for pain
- Compression Rotation test: (+) for pain or clicking
- Acromioclavicular Compression test: (–) for pain

Neurological Evaluation

- Dermatomes: C1 to C8 were normal
- Myotomes: C1 to C8 were normal
- No neurological symptoms reported subjectively

Discussion Questions

1. Based on the evaluation, what is the likely diagnosis?

2. What diagnostic test is most appropriate for this injury?

3. If the clinical evaluation remains the same the following day, is it appropriate to have the athlete attempt to throw pain free?

Resolution

The most likely diagnosis for this injury is a right shoulder labral injury. In this specific circumstance, the appropriate diagnostic test is a magnetic resonance arthrogram to evaluate the integrity of the labrum. In order for the athlete to resume throwing, the clinical evaluation would need to be unremarkable. In this instance, it would not be appropriate for the athlete to throw the following day if the clinical evaluation remained the same.

Notes:_____

_____

_____

_____

_____

_____

SCENARIO 11: BASEBALL COLLISION

During batting practice for the visiting team, 2 athletes collided going for a ball. Both players were lying on the ground. Player A was lying face up screaming and had a pain in his left knee, while Player B had low back pain and was lying face down not making much noise. The assistant coach was the first person to arrive at the scene. An athletic trainer was summoned to the scene to assess the situation and had to make a quick decision regarding which athlete he needed to assess first. The athletic trainer went to Player B to perform a primary survey for vital signs. The athletic trainer alerted the assistant baseball coach to go to Player A to calm him down and make sure Player A did not move. The athletic trainer assessed that Player B had no concussion and was alert but complaining of mild mid-back pain.

Discussion Questions

1. How would you manage the 2 athletes (Player A and Player B)?

2. What warning signs would you look for with Player B?

3. Define *shock* and describe its signs and symptoms. What is the earliest sign, and what is the latest?

Resolution

The athletic trainer assessed Player B's primary vital signs. Pulse and breathing were within the normal range. The athletic trainer performed sensory and motor tests for the cervical, thoracic, and lumbar spine. All tests were normal. Player B had no pain in deep inspiration, pain (5/10) along the left ribs posteriorly over ribs 8 to 12, and posterior left quadrant pain at 5/10. The athletic trainer took the blood pressure of Player B, which was 110/68. Player B was stable and stated he was feeling better. The athletic trainer had Player B slowly roll over to a supine position with the instruction to stop if it was painful. The athletic trainer asked the assistant coach to stay with Player B while he examined Player A. Player A stated that his knee pain was 2/10. Player A was able to move his knee with minimal discomfort. All examinations were normal for ligamentous and meniscal injuries. The athletic trainer continued to talk with Player B during the examination of Player A. Player B was pale, sweating, and answering questions slowly. The athletic trainer took Player B's blood pressure again, and it was 100/48. The athletic trainer determined that EMS should be summoned via campus police to transport Player B to the hospital and notified the visiting head baseball coach. The head baseball coach informed the athletic trainer that Player B's father would be arriving shortly to the field. The EMS and father arrived at the same time. The athletic trainer informed the father about what happened. Player B was transported to the local hospital. The athletic trainer continued to evaluate Player A, who had a contusion to his patella and was advised to use ice and compression and avoid physical activity. Later in the game, the visiting athletic trainer notified the athletic trainer that Player B had 4 broken ribs, a lacerated spleen, and a contusion to his left kidney.

*Notes:*_____

_____

_____

_____

_____

_____

Scenario 12: Concussion in Professional Baseball

A 27-year-old professional baseball player collided into the left field wall after making a diving catch. After colliding into the outfield wall (chain-link fence), he fell back onto the outfield warning track, then rolled onto his stomach showing the baseball to the field umpire. The athletic trainer ran onto the field to assess the athlete. The on-field assessment demonstrated that the player was conscious, alert, oriented, and sitting in a crouched position.

Discussion Questions

1. What would your on-field examination comprise? Begin with your subjective, objective, assessment, and plan.

2. What would your secondary examination in the athletic training room comprise? When would you refer the athlete to a doctor?

3. What subjective/objective findings will you need to clear the player back to competition? When should you administer the ImPACT test? When would you exert the athlete? If so, what kind of activities would you have him or her do?

Resolution

The athlete walked off of the field with assistance from the athletic trainer and the team's manager. He was re-examined by the medical staff in the athletic training room. The SCAT3 was administered, with a symptom score of 8. The remainder of the body was re-examined; he also sustained injuries to his right hand and left rib cage. He was also examined by the team's doctors. The doctors did not feel any diagnostic studies were needed and diagnosed the athlete with a mild concussion, a left rib cage contusion, and a right hand abrasion. The next day, the SCAT3 was repeated, with a symptom score of 0; the ImPACT computer test was administered, and the results were compared to his baseline test early in the season. The athlete was then exerted on a stationary bike, raising his heart rate up to 180 beats per minute. The activities did not cause any reoccurrence in symptoms. He was then cleared to participate in practice and play in the game.

*Notes:*_____

_____

_____

_____

_____

_____

SCENARIO 13: ALTERED PERSONALITY SIGNALS CONCUSSION IN A COLLEGIATE FOOTBALL PLAYER

During the third quarter of a college football playoff game, the visiting team's athletic trainer observed one of his players pacing the sideline. The score was close, and the player was noticeably fired up about the game. A few minutes earlier, he had made an outstanding tackle on a kickoff, and his teammates were quick to congratulate him. The player was a freshman who steadily improved during the season and made the playoff roster as a special team's player. The athletic trainer did not know the first-year player well and was not familiar with his personality. He rarely came into the athletic training room during the regular season. A few minutes later, after another special team's play, the athletic trainer observed the player parading the sideline with his fists clenched in the air. He slapped his helmet as if to self-motivate. The athletic trainer became suspicious of the player's behavior. Was this a normal level of intensity and enthusiasm for the player? Could it be a sign of a concussion? The athletic trainer talked to the player on the sideline. He asked whether he had sustained any hard hits to the head and if he felt concussed. The player assured the athletic trainer that he was okay. The athletic trainer took the player to the bench to assess him for a concussion. The player was cooperative, alert, and oriented. The athletic trainer completed the evaluation, with no findings of a concussion. The athletic trainer then checked with some teammates and an assistant coach to see if they thought that the player's sideline demeanor was normal. They commented on what a great game the player was having. Most of the teammates and the assistant coach were dismissive; however, one teammate believed that the behavior was atypical. Because the team physician did not travel with the team, the athletic trainer had to rely on assistance from the home team's physician. The athletic trainer sent an athletic training student to the other sideline to ask the home team's athletic trainer if their team physician would come to the visiting team bench to evaluate a player for a concussion. The home team's physician arrived at the visitor's bench within a few minutes and was briefed by the athletic trainer. The athletic trainer shared with the home team physician that the player's emotions on the sideline seemed unusually intense. The player's demeanor while on the bench had calmed. His behavior and interactions were normal during the physician's evaluation. The home team's physician completed his evaluation of the player and found no signs or symptoms of a concussion. The home team's physician decided to wait and re-evaluate the player again before making a return-to-play decision. In the interim, the athletic trainer continued to monitor the player.

Discussion Questions

1. How commonly do personality changes occur after a concussion?

2. What are some abnormal behaviors or emotions that an athlete with a concussion might display?

3. In addition to concussions, what other medical problems could cause a change in an athlete's personality?

Resolution

A close friend of the player and the player's father were among the fans at the football game. They were watching the game and observing the player from behind a fence separating the visiting team bench from the grandstands. They had noticed the player's hyped up sideline behavior in the third quarter and knew it was not consistent with his normal personality. A second team physician for the home team was not scheduled to work that day but had decided to come and watch part of the game. By chance, he was standing beside the player's father and the player's friend. The physician heard the father say that 2 years earlier, his son's personality had changed after he sustained a concussion in a high school football game. The 3 individuals connected with each other. They then caught the attention of the athletic trainer as he continued to monitor the player on the bench. The father confirmed with the athletic trainer that the player had been acting more emotionally on the sideline than normal and that it had happened previously in high school. The athletic trainer and the home team physician then substantiated that the sideline behavior that the athletic trainer had observed in the third quarter was not normal and was a sign of a concussion. The athletic trainer informed the coaches that the player would not return to play. The player was monitored by the athletic trainer for the remainder of the game. After the game ended, the home team physician re-evaluated the player. The player's personality change had resolved, but for the first time, he experienced other symptoms of a concussion. His new symptoms included a headache, feeling in a fog, and feeling irritable. The headache persisted for 48 hours, while the other 2 symptoms subsided within 30 minutes of onset. This situation was unique for 2 reasons: (1) along with the athletic trainer's unfamiliarity with the player, his personality change in the third quarter was suspicious but blended in with the heightened emotions and intensity displayed by many of the players during the playoff game and (2) when evaluated, the player interacted normally and had no other signs or symptoms of a concussion.

Notes:_____

_____

_____

_____

_____

_____

SCENARIO 14: CONFLICT RESOLUTION WITH AN INEXPERIENCED PHYSICIAN

This scenario involved a staff athletic trainer in his first year at a Division I institution coordinating the care for men's soccer. The athletic trainer had graduated from an accredited Post-Professional Master's Program in Athletic Training and was approximately 2 months into his first job working independently without supervision or direct mentoring. During a home soccer match, a defensive player sustained a knee injury during the first half that was not reported to the athletic trainer until half-time. Upon physical examination, there was mild extracapsular swelling around the lateral left knee joint line and a positive varus stress test between 20 to 30 degrees of knee flexion with significant laxity when compared bilaterally. The patient reported pain with running and cutting but no instances of functional instability in the first half after the injury occurred. Due to the concern for lateral collateral ligament rupture, the athletic trainer instructed the coach and the patient that he would not be available to play in the second half. The coach, noticing that the player completed the entire first half without obvious difficulty, did not agree with the decision and approached the sports medicine fellow (team physician), who was also covering the game. The team physician was just out of his residency and only 3 months into his sports medicine fellowship, with very little to no acute care sports medicine experience. The physician then examined the patient at the request of the head coach. Present for the evaluation during half-time were the physician, the patient, the head coach, and the athletic trainer. Following the conclusion of the examination, in which the physician concurred that his physical examination garnered the same results as the athletic trainer, the physician rendered his decision to the patient and the coach prior to discussing his findings with the athletic trainer.

Discussion Questions

1. Describe the roles and responsibilities of a resident or fellow (physician) who is working with an athletic trainer at an event.

2. What are limitations of a physician still in training?

3. What should the working relationship between an athletic trainer and a team physician be with regard to athletic coverage and emergency plan preparation?

Resolution

The team physician, without discussing with the staff athletic trainer first, disagreed with the decision of the athletic trainer. He told the patient and the coach that he believed that he could return to play for the second half due to the patient reporting no episodes of functional instability in the first half. Ultimately, the patient completed the second half with no reported increase in pain, no episodes of functional instability, and no apparent decrease in performance. A magnetic resonance image (MRI) obtained later in the season due to increased soreness in the patient's knee revealed a moderate partial tear of the lateral collateral ligament, with no other associated pathology. The patient never missed time due to this injury and, to date, has not required a procedure to address the knee injury.

Additional Resolution

If given the opportunity, I would have taken a firmer stance in my clinical decision, as I do not believe it was the correct call in the moment to let the patient return to activity. Furthermore, I would have appropriately educated the coach and the patient (perhaps after the game) about why I would attempt to overrule a physician. Although he was a physician, he was there in a learning capacity, and he was not well experienced in sports medicine. Finally, I would have spoken directly to the physician and made sure he understood my position. If he continued to disagree with me after our conversation, I would have asked him to consult with his supervising physician (the fellowship director) about the clinical decision that was made.

*Notes:*_____

_____

_____

_____

_____

SCENARIO 15: HYDROMYELIA/AMPLIFIED MUSCLE PAIN SYNDROME IN A FEMALE CROSS COUNTRY RUNNER

An 18-year-old female cross country runner presented with right femur pain since her race 2 days prior. She had an antalgic gait and a positive hip scour test. Because of her pain, she was placed on crutches. She was seen by the team orthopedic physician the next day (day 3). A knee MRI was ordered to rule out any knee pathology that he thought could be causing some of the symptoms. On day 10 (1 week later), she returned with the MRI and a significant increase in her symptoms. She was unable to bear weight, and her pain had drastically increased, specifically over her knee. On day 12 in rehabilitation, she could not straighten her knee without spastic motion. She had normal passive motion of 0 to 135 degrees, but as she extended to 55 degrees, she began to feel an increase in pain. At 35 degrees, her spasms became more pronounced and were exacerbated when a dorsiflexion component was added. On day 13, she was extremely sensitive to touch and complained that her sheet bothered her at night and that it was difficult to wear jeans, as they increased her pain. She was only able to extend her knee to -15 degrees due to pain. A desensitization program was initiated that consisted of rubbing a towel along her hypersensitive area.

Discussion Questions

1. What would cause her to be so sensitive in just one area?

2. Discuss the importance of follow-up evaluations in all injured patients.

3. What should be considered when symptoms that a patient is having do not match with traditional diagnosis or findings?

Resolution

The wife of the athlete's coach worked as a physical therapist at the Children's Hospital of Philadelphia (CHOP). She suggested that we discuss this case with the director of the Amplified Muscle Pain Syndrome (AMPS) program, one of the leading centers for this syndrome in the world. A video of her condition was sent to the AMPS program at CHOP. The director of the Physical Therapy Program felt that she clinically had AMPS but, unfortunately, could not be seen at CHOP because she was 18. A plan was sent and initiated for aggressive therapy to force motion and weightbearing and to continue her desensitization. The program director felt that, with its sudden onset, it should resolve faster than a normal presentation of AMPS.

In addition, for completeness, an MRI of her cervical, thoracic, and lumbar spine was ordered, and the results showed hydromyelia from T2 to T10. She was referred to a neurologist and placed on baclofen, an antispasmodic medicine, and acetazolamide, which was used to absorb fluids from the spinal cord. These are common medicines given prophylactically to mountain climbers at altitude.

She continued therapy for most of October and then did it on her own. She was walking normally by the end of October, and her symptoms had significantly improved; her hypersensitivity had waned and her motion had normalized. She followed up with her neurologist and a neurosurgeon, both of whom concluded that she did not need surgery. She returned to training the following summer and ran in cross country 1 year later.

*Notes:*_____

_____

_____

_____

_____

_____

SCENARIO 16: FACIAL FRACTURE IN MEN'S COLLEGIATE SOCCER PLAYER

A men's soccer player presented himself to the athletic trainer with facial discomfort following a blow to his face. He was charging the goal after the ball when the goalie came out and either punched his face with both fists—a typical goalie move to punch the ball away—or he collided with the goalie's shoulder.

He had significant pain over the left zygomatic arch and, from previous experience, the athletic trainer had a high suspicion of a fracture. The athlete also presented signs of a concussion. A smooth physical examination was completed to see if there was a possible entrapment of the eye muscles, and the examination was negative.

He was then sent to the emergency department, where a computed tomography scan was performed. The results showed that he had the following:

- Left inferior orbital fracture with comminuted fragments
- Nondisplaced fracture of the left zygomatic arch
- Nondisplaced fracture of the posterior maxillary wall sinus

Discussion Questions

1. What might you expect to see with your evaluation of an individual who sustained a blowout fracture?

2. Would you have completed a concussion evaluation? Why or why not?

3. Is the plastic face shield needed? Why or why not?

Resolution

After his return from the emergency department, a phone consultation was completed with an ophthalmic surgeon at the local hospital, who said that this situation usually called for collaboration with his service and oral/maxillofacial surgery. The student was from Connecticut and opted to have the surgery completed at home. Reduction of all fractures was completed, and titanium plates were placed for repair. He had an uncomplicated rehabilitation. Once he was cleared by his surgeon to begin activity, we followed our traumatic brain injury protocol. He was prescribed a plastic facial shield that was custom-made for his return to play.

*Notes:*_____

_____

_____

_____

_____

_____

SCENARIO 17: HIP INJURY IN A COLLEGE SWIMMER IN A WEIGHT ROOM

A 19-year-old female college swimmer had an episode in which her hip gave out on her in the weight room during a workout in the middle of the swimming season. Examination by the athletic trainer showed limited active and passive ROM in all directions due to pain. Passive ROM was hard to fully judge because the athlete was guarding. The athlete denied any numbness or tingling. She stated that she was unable to bear much weight on her affected side. She had a history of hip flexor strains during both years in college. Hip scouring test was positive. Pain was difficult to palpate because the athlete stated the pain was deep in the hip. She stated she felt a pop when the injury occurred. She was placed on crutches by the athletic trainer and was scheduled to see an orthopedic surgeon. She saw a hip specialist, who told her that she needed an MRI with contrast. The athletic trainer called every facility in the area that could perform the test to the specialist's exact specifications; the earliest appointment available for this athlete was 3 weeks away, and the physician would not allow her to do any lower body training until she saw the results of the MRI. When the athletic trainer updated the coach, he was upset that she could not train her lower body at all, especially because they were in the middle of the season. The coach felt that if she were a football or basketball athlete, the test would be performed that day. The athlete's parents emailed the athletic trainer and were concerned that the coach would try to push the athlete into the water before she was ready.

Discussion Questions

1. What is your plan of action for the athlete until she can get the MRI?

2. How do you handle the coach in this situation?

3. What do you say to the parents to keep them properly informed regarding this situation?

Resolution

I was able to explain the situation to the coach that the test was not just a standard MRI and that she needed an injection of dye into her hip joint before she had the images taken. Although we could have had a standard MRI done, they often miss a labrum tear. If the athlete had a labrum tear and we allowed her back into activity with this injury, she could do a lot of long-term damage to her hip. I also explained that we currently had a football player waiting for the same type of MRI for his shoulder and that he also had to wait 3 weeks. I started the athlete on pain-controlling modalities and basic hip ROM exercises that could be performed without pain. She also started some upper body lifting and upper body ergometer for cardio conditioning 4 to 5 times per week. I spoke to the parents about our plan of action for the athlete and let them know that the coach understood the ramifications of ignoring her restrictions and was now on board with the plan of care for the athlete. The athlete ended up having a labrum tear and had it repaired surgically once the semester was over. She had a successful rehabilitation and was cleared for full activity 4 months later.

Editor's Note

We cannot control the time lag we often experience in getting appointments for consultations or testing procedures. We can try to develop relationships with critical areas, such as radiology, to circumvent these delays, and the team physician can take the lead in establishing these relationships. I once had a good relationship with a local MRI facility that was established by providing tickets to games and other events. The relationship was so good that whenever I called for an appointment, the answer was, "When can he get here?"

*Notes:*_____

_____

_____

_____

_____

_____

SCENARIO 18: CONCUSSION FROM NOWHERE

You were at an away football game with your college team. One of the defensive backs sustained a head injury near the end of the game. You did not see the play, but his teammates alerted you to the fact that he was dazed and confused after sustaining a blow to the head. When you talked to him, he was suffering from retro- and anterograde amnesia. He denied losing consciousness. He stated that he had a bad headache. He denied any ringing in the ears, dizziness, light sensitivity, noise sensitivity, neck pain, numbness, and tingling in the extremities. Pupils were equal and reactive to light. Eye tracking was normal. Near and far vision were normal. Facial movement and sensation were within normal limits. Upper quarter screen—dermatomes and myotomes—were within normal limits. Rhomberg test was negative. Balance/coordination was normal. It was the end of the game when you completed the evaluation. You asked the home team's physician to evaluate the athlete, but he was an orthopedic physician and was not comfortable evaluating head injuries. You were 1.5 hours away from home in a rural area, with the closest hospital almost 1 hour away, and you knew from personal experience that it was a small hospital that was not the best. Even the visiting team athletic trainer did not recommend transfer to this facility. You were alarmed at the amnesia shown by the athlete as he did not know who you were and was unable to recognize his mother, who had made the trip to the game. You had one of his teammates help him change and shower. The teammate alerted you to the fact that the athlete became very emotional in the locker room because he did not recognize his mother. You were unsure if this injury was going to get any worse. His mother was worried about him but trusted your judgment for his treatment. His headache remained the same, about a 7/10. No other changes occurred in symptoms. It was about 30 minutes before the team was ready to leave. The ambulance had already left the stadium, and it could take some time before another ambulance arrived to transport the athlete to the emergency department if that is what you chose to do.

Discussion Questions

1. What were your athletic training options in this situation (at site and on the way home)?

2. How do you calm down the athlete's mother after you communicate with her about her son's medical situation?

3. What is your plan if the athlete gets worse on the way home?

Resolution

I decided that the best plan of action was to put the athlete on my bus in a seat with a responsible teammate to monitor him on the 90-minute trip home because he only had a headache, which was not increasing, and amnesia. I called our team physician, and he agreed with my plan. I explained to the mother that her son was currently stable and that although the amnesia was scary, he had no other worrisome symptoms. I felt that one of the local trauma hospitals was our best treatment option. If anything changed on the bus, we could call 911 and have him transported rapidly to a local trauma unit, but I was confident that he would be okay. The athlete slept the whole way home, and when he woke up at school, his headache decreased and he remembered everything. The athlete was symptom free 2 days later, passed ImPACT testing, and was gradually returned to activity following our return-to-play guidelines.

*Notes:*_____

_____

_____

_____

_____

SCENARIO 19: BROKEN SHOE?

A college running back took the handoff and broke through the line of scrimmage, at which point he was grabbed by a tackler around the foot and ankle. He did not go down but tried to get extra yardage while dragging the defensive tackler. Eventually, he was gang tackled by another member of the defense. The running back rolled into a seated position and grabbed the foot that was held by the first tackler with both hands. He then got up and jogged off to the sideline with a slight limp. As he approached the sideline, he told the coach that he broke the bottom of his shoe. The athletic trainer working the game approached the player, and the player also told him that his shoe was broken. The player flexed his toes in the shoe, and there was a visible shifting on the dorsum of the foot just below the laces. He was in no pain and sat down to remove his broken shoe. Once the shoe was removed and checked, it was determined that it was not damaged. The athletic trainer then removed the sock and began an evaluation on the affected foot. Upon inspection, there was no visible deformity, but the athlete was point tender on the dorsum of the foot with palpation. There was laxity in the mid-foot when stabilizing the foot at the ankle and lifting and depressing the metatarsals. The foot was immediately iced with a bag and a compression wrap. The player was fitted with crutches and sent to the emergency department for further medical evaluation.

Discussion Questions

1. What was the mechanism of injury to the foot?

2. Why did the athlete think that his shoe was broken?

3. What injury did the player sustain to his foot?

Resolution

The injury was determined to be a Lisfranc fracture upon further imaging and evaluation at the emergency department. Surgical intervention was the recommended medical procedure. The athlete recovered but decided not to return to football and focused on his studies at school.

*Notes:*_____

_____

_____

_____

_____

_____

SCENARIO 20: A HEATED DEBATE

I was working the finish line medical tent at a large spring marathon. A young woman was brought to the tent around the 4-hour mark. She had collapsed at the end of the race and appeared disoriented. Upon observing the initial entry and care for this woman, 2 concerning actions were taken. First, a rectal temperature and a blood sample (to assess blood sodium) were not taken, which would address 2 of the most highly suspected conditions (heat stroke and hyponatremia) for a woman in a marathon presenting with central nervous system dysfunction. Instead, an intravenous (IV) bag was administered in the absence of evaluating her blood sodium level. Despite having the ability to analyze a blood sample for sodium and glucose levels (considering she could have been hyponatremic or severely hypoglycemic), this was not done prior to administering this treatment.

Second, when her level of consciousness did not improve, the decision was made to transport her to the hospital. At this point, neither hyponatremia nor heat stroke had been appropriately ruled in or out. The steps of obtaining blood sodium and a rectal temperature were presented in the marathon medical meeting earlier that day, outlined in the algorithms for treating a patient with central nervous system dysfunction, and considered the protocol that should be followed for this race. Given the implications of any delay in treatment for these conditions, I decided to propose further evaluation, specifically by obtaining a rectal temperature to quickly determine if exertional heat stroke was the culprit as it is the only accurate option to obtain body temperature in an exercising individual.

My suggestion of taking a rectal temperature was met with great resistance. My largest concern was that she would not be cooled within an appropriate amount of time (30 minutes) to prevent sequelae or death if she was suffering heat stroke. Similarly, if she was hyponatremic, she would need hypertonic saline as soon as possible.

Discussion Questions

1. What are the top 3 conditions you suspect upon initial evaluation, and how would you rule those in or out? What would your initial steps be for this athlete given her presentation and immediate exercise history?

2. If you did not have access to a rectal thermometer or ability to analyze blood glucose/sodium, what would your next step be?

3. What is your immediate priority for this patient considering the condition(s) you most likely suspect?

Resolution

My suggestion to take a rectal temperature was dismissed, and the patient was transported to the hospital to my great dismay. Furthermore, following this incident, I was informed that I had offended the other medical providers in charge of this woman's treatment and I was not to volunteer for the medical tent or return in subsequent years. Although I am disappointed I am not able to return to the race, I do not regret intervening on behalf of a patient with the best interest of the patient (ultimately her life) at heart.

*Notes:*_____

_____

_____

_____

_____

_____

SCENARIO 21: STRESS FRACTURE IN FEMUR OF COLLEGE DISTANCE RUNNER

A men's track and field distance runner presented with left thigh pain that had been increasing over 1 week with training. The athlete now had pain with walking. He was seen in an injury clinic with an orthopedic resident 4 days after the pain started. During the evaluation, the physician found that there had been no change in the training schedule and no prior injuries, and hill running was most painful. The athlete's medical history was unremarkable.

On physical examination, there was pain with deep palpation at the left proximal thigh. He presented with full pain-free active ROM of the left hip. The athlete had pain with resisted left hip flexion and pain at his proximal thigh with percussion at the calcaneus. The athlete had no palpable masses, a negative straight leg raise test, and a negative log roll, and he was neurovascularly intact.

The athlete was placed nonweightbearing on crutches. He was sent for x-rays of his left hip and femur. The radiologist report revealed no fracture, subluxation, or osseous lesion. There was prominence of the soft tissues of the mid to proximal left thigh. The head orthopedic surgeon ordered an MRI of the left hip without contrast. The radiology report indicated bone marrow edema and periostitis in the mid diaphysis of the left femur, consistent with a stress reaction. The radiologist reported that early infection or a neoplasm would have a similar appearance. The athlete continued to be nonweightbearing while more tests were ordered.

Discussion Questions

1. What other imaging tests could have been used and why?

2. Before the athlete started to run again, discuss 2 functional assessments you could have done.

3. Describe a return-to-run program and how to safely progress the athlete.

Resolution

The head orthopedic surgeon ordered a bone scan to confirm a stress fracture diagnosis and rule out neoplasm. The bone scan was 2 weeks after the athlete reported thigh pain, and the findings were consistent with a stress fracture. The radiologist indicated that there was increased osseous uptake along the medial posterior cortex of the left femur.

The athlete continued to be nonweightbearing for 4 weeks. At 4 weeks, he was cleared to do nonimpact conditioning and core exercises that did not increase his pain. Six weeks after the injury was reported, the athlete continued to have pain and remained nonweightbearing on the crutches. Our primary care sports medicine fellow ordered vitamin D_2 and vitamin D_3 laboratory tests. After the laboratory results were reviewed, he was placed on a calcium supplement daily and 5000 units daily of vitamin D_3.

At 8 weeks postinjury, the athlete reported no pain with walking or palpation and was cleared to begin running again. For 2 weeks, he was advised to run 3 days per week. The team physician wanted him to begin with 20 minutes and increase to 30 minutes over the 3 days. He was allowed to bike longer for cardiovascular training. Over the course of 4 weeks, he gradually increased his running time. The athlete followed the physician's protocol and did not increase his mileage more than 10% in 1 week.

At 6 weeks of his return-to-running program, the athlete reported that he was starting to have pain with running. A follow-up visit was scheduled with the head orthopedic surgeon, and a follow-up MRI was ordered. The MRI indicated a healing stress fracture of the left femur. At the time of this writing, the athlete was advised to discontinue running for 3 more weeks. In 1 month, he could begin a slow return-to-running program and return for follow-up as needed.

Additional Resolution

I would have ordered more laboratory tests. Because the physician was ruling out a cancer diagnosis, a complete metabolic panel and complete blood count would have given more information. A referral to a nutritionist may have been beneficial to help with the athlete's calcium deficiency.

Notes:_____

_____

_____

_____

_____

_____

SCENARIO 22: RIGHT SERRATUS ANTERIOR AVULSION FROM LOWER RIB INSERTION

A defensive end for the football team came to the athletic training room reporting pain along the lateral aspect of his right ribs. The athlete told the athletic trainer that he was performing a one-arm dumbbell press and felt a cramp in the area of discomfort. The athlete said he continued to work through it but that he had trouble moving his upper extremity in all ROMs. He was performing one-arm exercises due to recovering from left posteroinferior labral repair performed the previous January.

Upon evaluation, the athletic trainer noted no obvious deformity, no ecchymosis, and tenderness to palpation over the lateral aspect of the chest wall most noted along ribs 6 to 8. The athlete was able to play his position but was required to do right shoulder/serratus anterior strengthening. In a game 12 days later, the athlete felt a pop while trying to block a punt but denied any other trauma. The athlete had no difficulty breathing, numbness, or other systemic complaints in his medical history and had no known allergies. On examination, the athlete had full but painful ROM. Scapulothoracic dyskinesis was noted on the right side, but no winging or elevation was noticeable. The athlete was unable to perform a wall push-up. He had equal strength bilaterally with no instability. Other parts of the physical examination were within normal limits. Chest posteroanterior/lateral and right-sided rib x-rays showed no acute fracture; cardiopulmonary views were noted. Soft tissue swelling was seen along the right lateral chest wall. An MRI of the scapula/chest wall showed a complete detachment of the inferior one-half of the right-sided serratus anterior muscle from the rib attachments.

The athlete was treated with oral medications. The motions that caused pain were restricted while he performed rehabilitative exercises with the athletic trainer focusing on rotator cuff and periscapular strengthening. The athlete had a surgical consult and was placed in an S3 (scapulothoracic brace).

Discussion Questions

1. What measures could have been taken before the athlete felt it necessary to only do one-arm workouts in the weight room?

2. What are some of the rehabilitation exercises that the athlete could do to strengthen this muscle before return to play?

3. Describe a return-to-play program and how to safely progress the athlete.

Resolution

After about 2 weeks of aggressive rehabilitation with the athletic trainer, the athlete was able to return to participation in football. The rehabilitation that the athlete was asked to perform focused on the rotator cuff, scapular stabilizers, and proprioception of the right shoulder and chest wall. Rehabilitation improved the athlete's ROM, strength, and shoulder dyskinesia. The athlete was required to wear the brace to play and was able to return to play after missing only 2 football games. He was able to play in the remaining 3 games of the regular season and had no residual symptoms.

Additional Resolution

The changes that I think needed to be made would probably have been to communicate better with the athlete when he felt the need to only work one arm due to the pain in his surgically repaired shoulder. It probably would have served him better to pull him out of the weight room and place him back in rehabilitation. After the athlete suffered the right strained serratus anterior, I would have also rehabilitated it more aggressively to possibly prevent this injury from happening.

Notes:_____
_____
_____
_____
_____
_____

SCENARIO 23: COLLEGIATE SOCCER KNEE INJURY

You are an athletic trainer covering a collegiate soccer match. The goalkeeper made a diving save and came to rest in a side-lying fetal position facing the field. An opposing player who was sprinting toward the goal was unable to stop in time to avoid the goalkeeper and slid feet-first into her shins. The goalkeeper immediately began rolling around clutching her left knee in obvious significant pain. You arrived at her side but could get no useful information from her due to her distress. You saw no obvious deformity and carefully took down her sock. There were distinct cleat marks over her proximal anterior and anterolateral tibia just above her shin guard. The skin was not broken but was already slightly swollen and discolored around the cleat marks. When she calmed down, the athlete said that her pain was throughout the knee and shin and she thought she felt a pop when the opposing player's cleats hit her leg.

Discussion Questions

1. What type of injury evaluation should be conducted on the field?

2. Under what conditions will the athlete require splinting on the field?

3. Keeping in mind the obvious trauma to the proximal anterolateral shin, what serious condition might later develop?

Resolution

There was no apparent deformity of the tibia, but the athlete was guarding the knee too much to allow ligamentous laxity testing. She was able to bear some weight and was helped off the field with a significant limp. You immobilized her knee, and she was transported by cart to the team facility, where an x-ray of her tibia was negative for fracture. She was later found to have a grade 3 posterior cruciate ligament injury, and after several weeks of treatment and rehabilitation, she underwent ligament reconstruction surgery.

*Notes:*_____

_____

_____

_____

_____

SCENARIO 24: UPPER EXTREMITY EFFORT THROMBOSIS IN A VOLLEYBALL PLAYER

A 22-year-old female volleyball player presented to the athletic training room after practice with left forearm tightness and pain in the left bicep. She stated that she felt like she was not getting any blood flow into her arm. The pain gradually increased and did not go away until after she quit working out. There was no previous history of injury, and the athlete was right-hand dominant. Physical examination revealed swelling and discoloration in the left arm, with obvious bulging of veins in the left arm. Shoulder and elbow ROM were normal; shoulder abduction to 90 degrees caused a decrease in pulse. Adson test was negative but no other special tests were performed. Neurological examination indicated normal myotomes and reflexes but decreased sensation over C6 to C7. Pulses were equal and capillary refill was brisk. No immediate treatment was warranted per a verbal order from the team physician.

The athlete presented 2 days later with the same symptoms and was referred to the emergency department. X-rays were normal, and she was discharged and referred to a specialist for further evaluation.

Discussion Questions

1. What other components of the physical examination (ie, soft tissue tests) could have been completed by the athletic trainer?

2. Based on the information in the scenario, what anatomical structures could have caused the effort thrombosis?

3. What types of diagnostic tests would need to be ordered to further evaluate this athlete? What would you expect to find with each test?

Resolution

An upper extremity venous ultrasound revealed a large completely occluding thrombus in the left subclavian vein. The athlete was admitted to the hospital for an angioplasty, which was unsuccessful. Heparin IV was started and was converted to subcutaneous injections upon discharge. One month later, the athlete underwent resection of the first rib and costoclavicular ligament, anterior scalenectomy, and decompression of the axillary subclavian vein. She was discharged 4 days later with instructions for rehabilitation with the athletic trainer. Full strength and ROM were restored; however, the athlete chose not to return to volleyball the next season.

Additional Resolution

The initial assessment should have warranted a referral to the emergency room. The athlete continued to practice for 2 more days before receiving advanced care. Also, postsurgical rehabilitation should have focused on the psychosocial aspect more in hopes of encouraging return to play.

Notes:_____

_____

_____

_____

_____

_____

SCENARIO 25: *STAPHYLOCOCCUS* INFECTION IN A COLLEGIATE FOOTBALL PLAYER

A 22-year-old male football athlete presented to the athletic trainer with generalized pain in his left shoulder. The athlete was the right-hand–dominant starting center on the varsity football team. The team was in the middle of preseason practices. The weather was hot and humid, with the temperature in the mid-90s and the humidity around 80%. The athletic trainer evaluated the athlete's shoulder on the field. There was no history of a singular episode that the athlete remembered. He reported vague, aching, dull pain, which was not in a consistent area. There was no specific pain on palpation and no positive results on any special tests. His strength was within normal limits. A diagnosis of a contusion with muscle soreness was presumed, and the athlete continued to practice. The pain resolved within 48 hours. Several days later, the athlete reported pain in his left wrist with no specific mechanism of injury, which also resolved over a short time. Two days prior to the first game, the athlete reported nonspecific left knee pain. There was no history of a traumatic event that the athlete could remember. He had undergone anterior cruciate ligament reconstruction on the left knee 1 year previously. Evaluation of the knee was inconclusive and did not seem related to the previous anterior cruciate ligament surgery. The next day, after a light practice, the athlete was noticed limping. When confronted by the athletic trainer, he stated his left calf was tight and sore. Upon examination, the athletic trainer noticed the calf was markedly swollen with pitting edema and was hot to the touch. With further questioning, the athlete stated he had been taking care of an ingrown toenail on his left, great toe. Examination showed redness, swelling, and pus around the nail, with warmth in the foot and lower leg. The athlete had a fever of 101°F.

Discussion Questions

1. What are the signs and symptoms of a localized infection?

2. What are the signs and symptoms of a systemic infection?

3. Which antibiotics are indicated for a staph infection?

Resolution

The athlete was referred to the team internist. He was diagnosed with a systemic *Staphylococcus* infection from the ingrown toenail. He was admitted to the hospital and immediately placed on IV antibiotics. Diagnostic imaging showed an abscess in the left calf. He was taken to the operating room the next day, where an incision and drainage of the left calf was performed. It was believed that the infection colonized near the surgical hardware and tracked to the calf. Systemic embolization of the bacteria may have caused the migrating joint pain he experienced. The athlete remained hospitalized for 10 days. He received IV antibiotics for the next 6 weeks. He was unable to return to football for the remainder of the season.

Additional Resolution

The athlete was not typically a complainer. He was a senior and was very dedicated. We thought it was strange that all of his complaints were on the left side and had no real mechanisms of injury. Our mindset focused on orthopedic injuries and we should have looked for other causes earlier.

Notes:_____

_____

_____

_____

_____

_____

SCENARIO 26: MULTIPLE SCLEROSIS IN A COLLEGIATE GOLFER

A 22-year-old golfer came to the athletic training room with right-sided facial numbness. The numbness had begun at his right ear and increased in area over 2 days. On the morning in question, he awoke with right arm and hand paresthesia that improved over 45 minutes. He denied other unusual symptoms or significant past medical problems. He denied any signs or symptoms of a cold or viral illness. He had been playing a normal amount of golf with no unusual stressors. A head, eyes, ears, nose, and throat examination was normal, with the exception of a Rinne test that lateralized to the left ear. Eye examination was normal, with acceptable visual acuity and normal pupillary reaction to light and accommodation. Cranial nerves II to XII were otherwise normal. Due to the numbness in his right arm and hand, an upper body orthopedic assessment was performed. All special tests were negative, and his ROM and strength were within normal limits. A mild sensory deficit was noted on his right arm and hand. The athlete was restricted from physical activity and referred to a medical specialist. He continued to experience numbness in his right arm and hand and later started having numbness in all extremities prior to his appointment with the specialist.

Discussion Questions

1. What type of medical specialist should this patient see for his symptoms, and what special tests should be prescribed?

2. What is the long-term prognosis for this athlete?

3. What additional symptoms will start to appear in the future?

Resolution

The athlete was examined by the neurologist. He was prescribed aspirin. An MRI of the brain was ordered. The initial differential diagnoses included Bell's palsy, meningitis, migraine headaches, stroke, multiple sclerosis, amyotrophic lateral sclerosis, and Guillain-Barré syndrome. The MRI findings included numerous oval-shaped T2/Flair hyperintensities in periventricular and deep white matter within the frontal, parietal, and temporal lobes bilaterally. The overall constellation of findings was most consistent with manifestations of a demyelinating disease related to multiple sclerosis. The athlete was started on copaxone, a self-injection of 20 mg once per day, which he currently continues. He was cleared to play golf by the neurologist with no restrictions 3 weeks after the initial presentation. Once released to activity, he continued to practice golf. He began competing in golf tournaments 6 months after his diagnosis.

*Notes:*_____

_____

_____

_____

_____

_____

SCENARIO 27: CERVICAL SPINE INJURY IN A COLLEGIATE FOOTBALL PLAYER

During a spring practice session, which was being held in our indoor practice facility due to inclement weather, a receiver was running a pass pattern when he lost his balance and ran head-first into the padded wall. The athletic trainer witnessed the impact from 10 yards away and noted that it was an axial load mechanism. Upon reaching the downed athlete, he was noted to be conscious, alert, and complaining of tingling all over his body. His head was immobilized by the assistant athletic trainer while a thorough secondary survey was completed. He had no loss of consciousness and had patent airway, his pulse was strong, and his blood pressure was within normal limits. He had no motor or sensory activity in any extremity. It was determined that he had a significant spinal cord injury, and EMS was activated. The EAP was then followed. After carefully removing the facemask, the medical staff immobilized the athlete, with his helmet and shoulder pads in place, while awaiting EMS arrival. The athletic trainer accompanied the athlete to the emergency department to assist with care decisions and with equipment removal when appropriate. The athlete was immediately taken to a trauma bay in the emergency department. While giving the attending physician a report, the athletic trainer turned around to note that the emergency department staff had removed the equipment very quickly and with no particular method. The athlete was then placed in a cervical collar, underwent radiology testing, and was transferred to the neuro intensive care unit.

Discussion Questions

1. What is the athletic trainer's role in the emergency department in a situation like this?

2. What are your thoughts and philosophies on equipment removal at the scene vs at the hospital?

3. How can the EAP be adapted to prevent another situation like this from occurring?

Resolution

The athlete was diagnosed with a complete spinal cord rupture at C4-C5 and is a quadriplegic. He was hospitalized for an extended period of time and was then transferred to a rehabilitation facility.

Additional Resolution

This situation was handled appropriately until the emergency room staff removed the equipment with no method or forethought. This was one of the main reasons that the athletic trainer accompanied the athlete to the hospital. The athletic trainer should have been more aware of what was going on in the emergency room and made it clear that he would assist in the removal of the equipment.

Notes:_____

_____

_____

_____

_____

_____

3

Domain III
Immediate and Emergency Care

SCENARIO 1: MANAGING HEAD INJURIES IN A WRESTLING MATCH

During a match, a high school wrestler collided head to head with another wrestler while attempting a takedown. He was winning by a score of 6 to 5. The official stopped the match to have the wrestler checked out by the athletic trainer. No illegal move was called and no type of misconduct penalty was awarded to either wrestler, so if either wrestler could not continue, a forfeit would be awarded to the able wrestler, as well as 6 team points, possibly costing the other team the match.

The athletic trainer was given 1 minute and 30 seconds of injury time for an evaluation. Upon examination, the wrestler insisted he was fine, but he looked a little out of it. The athlete reported no symptoms other than some blurred vision in the eye on the side of the collision. The athlete passed all tests and answered all questions. Meanwhile, the coaches were giving instructions while the athletic trainer was trying to assess the wrestler.

Discussion Questions

1. How would you handle this situation?

2. What special tests would you focus on?

3. What history questions would you ask?

Gorse KM, Feld F, Blanc RO, eds.
*Athletic Training Case Scenarios:
Domain-Based Situations and Solutions* (pp 89-140).
© 2016 Taylor & Francis Group.

Resolution

Wrestling is easily one of the hardest sports in which to manage injuries during competition, especially head injuries. Many symptoms can take hours or days to manifest. Athletic trainers are given 1 minute and 30 seconds to make a return-to-play decision. In this situation, the athlete was allowed to continue due to (1) the athletic trainer knowing the athlete and his personality and (2) because the blurred vision was only in one eye and was near the site of impact.

Additional Resolution

There should be a separate injury time for head injuries. Five minutes is currently allotted for blood time and 1 minute and 30 seconds is allotted for all other injuries. Five minutes for a head injury should be allotted due to the possible delay in symptoms. Also, during that time, coaches should not be allowed to coach their wrestler. If possible, no contact should be allowed if an athletic trainer or physician is present.

Editor's Note

This demonstrates why athletic trainers must work together to effect rule changes that are in the interests of athlete safety. One athletic trainer asking for a rule change will be ignored, but if many athletic trainers get their state organization to lobby for a rule change, it will be harder for governing athletic organizations to ignore the request. This is especially true if team physicians follow suit and start to demand changes. There is strength in numbers, but it takes one to get the ball rolling.

Notes:_____

_____

_____

_____

_____

_____

SCENARIO 2: MANAGEMENT OF MULTIPLE INJURED ATHLETES

An athletic trainer was covering a college women's soccer team during a training session. During the last 5 minutes of the session while the team was scrimmaging 11 vs 11, one of the athletes was sprinting into the box with the ball when the goalkeeper came out and they collided. As they slid into each other, the goalkeeper's knee made contact with the field player's jaw. As the athletic trainer approached, the goalkeeper was rolling around yelling in pain and holding her knee while the field player was lying flat on her back, eyes wide open and unconscious.

The athletic trainer approached the unconscious field player first and called her name while tapping her on the shoulder with no response. Emergency medical services (EMS) was notified. Next, as the athletic trainer began to check the airway, breathing, and circulation, blood started to come out of the athlete's mouth. The athletic trainer stabilized her head and neck while a coach and 2 other athletes assisted with rolling the injured athlete onto her side. The athlete regained consciousness and was stabilized until EMS arrived.

Discussion Questions

1. What is triage? Discuss the classifications used for prioritizing care for multiple patients.

2. What would be the athletic trainer's next steps in managing the injured field player?

3. What would be the athletic trainer's steps to manage the injured goalkeeper?

Resolution

When EMS arrived, they spine boarded the field player and transported her to the emergency department. She was evaluated by a physician and underwent some diagnostic testing. The field player was diagnosed with a fractured mandible, 2 dislocated teeth, a tongue laceration, and a concussion. Her jaw was wired shut for 6 to 8 weeks. She eventually recovered and returned to play soccer.

The goalkeeper had her knee evaluated by the athletic trainer. She presented with pain and tenderness over the lateral and inferior portion of her left patella with moderate swelling. She was full weightbearing, had full range of motion (ROM), and manual muscle testing was within normal limits. Ligamentous and meniscal examination was negative, and neurological examination was intact. It was determined that the goalkeeper suffered a significant lateral knee contusion. She was treated with cryotherapy and ROM exercises. The contusion eventually resolved, and she returned to play without limitations.

*Notes:*_____

_____

_____

_____

_____

_____

SCENARIO 3: KNEE DISLOCATION
IN COLLEGE FOOTBALL GAME

A college football linebacker was forced into hyperextension in his right knee while making a tackle. The athletic trainer arrived on the field, and the student athlete presented with obvious deformity of the right knee as well as noticeable pain and distress. The athlete was conscious and interactive. The athlete was rolled to a supine position while supporting his right leg. His shoe and ankle tape were then removed as the athletic trainer began his evaluation. The athletic trainer determined that there was an intermittent dorsalis pedis pulse, no posterior tibialis pulse, and no ankle or great toe dorsiflexion, but that he was able to plantarflex both and had no sensation over the dorsum of the foot. The athletic trainer then activated their emergency action plan (EAP) and called for EMS to prepare to transport the athlete. Prior to transporting the student athlete to the nearest Level I trauma emergency department, the leg was immobilized in a full-length vacuum splint, and the athlete was spine boarded for transport as well as for the potential risk of shock. The athlete was transported from the field in less than 5 minutes after the injury and arrived at the emergency department for relocation of the knee within 18 minutes of the mechanism of injury.

Discussion Questions

1. Why was it important to remove the athlete's shoe, sock, and tape at the beginning of the evaluation by the athletic trainer and physician?

2. The athlete was spine boarded for transport due to the risk of shock. What are the signs and symptoms of shock?

3. What are the long-term concerns with a peroneal neuropathy?

Resolution

The athletic trainer and team physician traveled with the student athlete to the emergency department, where the orthopedic surgeon reduced the dislocation and reassessed his distal pulses and strength. The athlete's knee was determined to be grossly unstable, at which point an external fixation was surgically applied. The student athlete was admitted for pain control and gait training before beginning the surgical plan of reconstructing the ruptured soft tissue structures.

*Notes:*_____

_____

_____

_____

_____

_____

SCENARIO 4: COOPERATION FROM OPPOSING COACHES AND POOR EMERGENCY MEDICAL SERVICES RESPONSE TIME

During a city league midget football game on an away field with 9 and 10 year olds playing, one of your players went down on the opposite side of the field. When you got to him, he was grasping his left arm and crying hard. Inspection showed a deep open slash from his elbow to his wrist, which made the officials and opposing coaches gasp. The athlete was alert, was oriented, could move all of his joints, and had no other pain complaints. When you walked the player over to the sideline, the wound was only bleeding superficially, and the player seemed in control of himself. His mother then came onto the field. Fortunately, she was calm. You explained to them both that he needed to be seen in the emergency department. The mother decided to wait for an ambulance to take them. You called 911 and sent them out to the street to wait. (City midget football leagues do not have ambulances at the playing fields.)

Discussion Questions

1. In this scenario, why would it be important to cover the wound on the field?

2. After attending to the player, what would be your next actions, and why would they be important?

3. If the opposing coach is unwilling to stop play until you have inspected the field, what would your actions be?

Resolution

The player had 39 total sutures. His mother refused to let him return to play after he healed. The officials and the entire midget football organization now allow the athletic trainer to request stop play when there are safety issues and/or when injuries occur. The city 911 cannot provide immediate response times unless there is a life-or-death scenario.

*Notes:*_____

_____

_____

_____

_____

_____

SCENARIO 5: SPECTATOR AT AN ATHLETIC EVENT

It was a very hot and humid home game day. Midway through the third quarter, one of the security people at the field came over to your sideline and told you that a spectator needed assistance. You went to the bleacher area and found that the spectator was a young mother of a player on the visiting team who was more than 8 months pregnant and was feeling sick. Her pulse was rapid and thread, she was sweating profusely, and she told you she just felt "funny." You suggested that she should go to the emergency department to get checked, but she refused. She stated that there was no other family at the game with her.

Discussion Questions

1. What would you do if you heard there was a medical emergency with a spectator?

2. What do you do if an injured/ill spectator continued to ignore your suggestions?

3. Are you responsible for the health and safety of spectators at events? Are you responsible for them if they do not accept your suggestions?

Resolution

After calling 911 and then returning to the bleachers to check on the pregnant woman, she was gone, and bystanders did not know where she had gone.

*Notes:*_____

_____

_____

_____

_____

_____

SCENARIO 6: SPINE BOARDING OF A DIVER IN A POOL

A 21-year-old female diver sustained a laceration to her forehead on the diving board at the initiation of her entry. An athletic trainer and an athletic training student were summoned to the pool deck from the athletic training room. While still in the pool, the athlete was holding pressure to her forehead over the injury site. The head diving coach was lying prone at the side of the pool deck stabilizing the athlete's head and neck at the level of her mastoid processes and was encouraged to continue to do so during the initial evaluation. The athlete was conscious; was breathing; had equal, round, and reactive pupils; and was responsive to questions.

The athletic trainer assessed the level of blood and began the initial assessment. The athletic trainer placed gloves on and asked the athlete to place a piece of gauze under her hand and to keep pressure over the open wound. During this time, the athletic trainer inquired of the athlete's symptoms; she complained primarily of head pain at the injury site. The athletic trainer then palpated the athlete's cervical vertebrae, with pain reported upon palpation of C2 and C3. The athlete reported no neurological symptoms. The athlete stated that she dove a tower practice the previous day, which typically made her neck sore; however, due to the presence of central cervical spine pain with palpation and the mechanism of direct contact with the diving board, the athletic trainer initiated the spine boarding EAP. The student athletic trainer was asked to call EMS and retrieve the spine board. A lifeguard on duty was also available to help.

Because the athlete was upright, she first needed to be moved into a supine position. The lifeguard who entered the pool was asked to position himself below the athlete to support the weight of her body as she had previously been holding herself up with only one arm. The athlete, with the assistance of the coach and teammate, was then gently transitioned into a supine position parallel to the wall. The spine board was then submerged perpendicular to the water, parallel to the side of the pool, and was then allowed to float perpendicular to the wall underneath the athlete. The spider straps and head blocks were then attached and secured to the board. A rigid cervical collar was attempted to be used on the athlete, but it did not fit properly. The local EMS arrived and assisted in the removal of the athlete from the pool on the spine board.

Discussion Questions

1. How does an EAP help in this swimming/diving situation?

2. What special protocol should athletic trainers use in swimming pool emergency situations?

3. When placing the injured athlete on the spine board, describe proper positioning of all rescuers in the water and on the pool deck.

Resolution

The athlete was transported via EMS to the emergency care facility, where she received x-rays and a computed tomography (CT) scan. No cervical spine pathology was present. Closure of the laceration on her forehead was achieved with 25 sutures prior to discharge. The athlete was promptly seen the following morning by the team physician. At initial evaluation, the athlete had described primarily head pain at the site of the injury and denied other concussion symptoms when asked; however, approximately 12 hours later, the athlete presented with a multitude of concussion symptoms. She was held from participation until the resolution of her symptoms, at which time she chose to discontinue diving.

Additional Resolution

The rigid cervical collar on the pool deck was not adjustable and did not fit this particular athlete. Following this incident, the certified athletic trainer promptly ordered an adjustable cervical collar to be attached to the spine board on the pool deck.

Notes:_____

_____

_____

_____

_____

_____

SCENARIO 7: ON-FIELD FIBULAR FRACTURE

A high school football player sustained a direct blow to the lateral aspect of the lower leg during a Friday night football game. The athlete displayed an antalgic gait and minimal discomfort as he came off the field. He reported a cramping sensation along the lateral compartment of his lower leg but stated he had no pain and wished to return to the field. The athletic trainer told the athlete that he needed to be evaluated first and instructed him to lay down on the sideline to be evaluated for injury. Upon examination, the athletic trainer noticed no deformity, muscle spasm, or tonus but did notice moderate crepitus with initial palpation. The palpation caused no pain, and the initial crepitus replicated with additional testing. Throughout the evaluation, the athlete continued to argue that he was fine and wished to return to play. The evaluation showed a slight decrease in ROM and strength with eversion. Compression and percussion tests were negative. However, the athletic trainer sensed the initial crepitus could be an issue and called for the team physician. He conveyed his findings and concerns to the team physician, whose evaluation noticed some mild initial crepitus that did not replicate with additional testing.

Discussion Questions

1. Based on the athlete's symptoms and hit he incurred, would you return the athlete to competition? What is your reasoning for making this decision?

2. Once activated, what is the role of each member of the EAP, and what information should be conveyed to those involved?

3. How could the communication between the parent and on-call orthopedist been improved?

Resolution

After a brief discussion, it was determined that the athlete would be transported to the hospital for x-rays. The EMS was brought over and instructed to splint the leg and transport the athlete to the hospital. The EMS, seeing the athlete was in no distress and showed no obvious sign of fracture, argued that splinting was unnecessary. The team physician intervened and demanded they splint the leg prior to transport. At this time, the athlete's mother came down from the stands and was informed that there was the possibility of a fibular fracture and that he was being sent to the hospital for x-rays and further evaluation. The athlete was transported to the hospital, where he was evaluated by the on-call orthopedic physician. His evaluation in the hospital was similar to the on-field evaluation. He showed no distress, crepitus, or sign of fracture. The orthopedic initially stated there was no need for an x-ray. The athlete's mother argued that the athletic trainer and team physician both showed concern for fracture and demanded an x-ray be taken. The orthopedist relented and ordered the x-ray which displayed a comminuted and spiral fracture of the fibula. The athlete was then casted and placed on crutches.

Additional Resolution

I would have ensured that our team physician contacted the hospital in advance to convey his findings to the on-call orthopedist. This may have saved time and prevented the parent from having to argue with the hospital staff about obtaining the x-ray. I also would have ensured that we had our own splinting equipment on the field so that we could have splinted the athlete immediately and prevented any confrontation with the EMS on site.

Notes:
_____

_____

_____

_____

_____

_____

SCENARIO 8: UNUSUAL SUBDURAL HEMATOMA

An athlete was hit awkwardly in the chest during a catch/tackle drill. Toward the end of the drill, the athletic trainer noticed that the athlete was not participating in the drill. When asked by the athletic trainer how he was feeling, he stated that he had the wind knocked out of him and he would be okay. Otherwise, the athlete appeared normal and responsive. He did not finish the drill because practice was ending. He did not participate in post-practice conditioning. He was asked to return to the athletic training room after practice.

Following practice (approximately 10 minutes later), he entered the athletic training room and stated that he did not feel right and asked if he could be examined. As he sat on the table, he fell to the floor unconscious in seizure with a positive fencing response. As the seizure subsided, the athlete was stabilized and the EMS was called to the scene. Within 1 minute, the athlete was responsive, although confused. The athlete continued respirations without difficulty, and vital signs remained normal.

It was decided not to put him on a spine board at that time. The athletic training room was cramped, and not enough people were available. The athletic trainer waited for EMS to arrive and the athlete was transported to the hospital for further evaluation.

Discussion Questions

1. What are 3 potential differential diagnoses for this scenario?

2. How would you stabilize an athlete who is seizing in an enclosed area?

3. What information is important to document concerning seizure activity?

Resolution

The athlete was evaluated by a CT scan and was found to have a subdural hematoma. He was observed for 2 days, and another CT scan showed that the hematoma was not increasing in size. It was decided not to do surgery and to let the hematoma resolve on its own. He had concussion symptoms that resolved and had no other complications related to the hematoma. He was not permitted to return to collision sports and chose not to return to sports.

Notes:_____

_____

_____

_____

_____

_____

SCENARIO 9: BLUNT ABDOMINAL TRAUMA IN A SOCCER GOALKEEPER

An athletic training student at a small, private, very rural college was assigned to the men's soccer team and worked under the head athletic trainer. During a soccer game, the goalkeeper on their team collided with a forward on the other team while going for the ball in the air. The goalkeeper jumped up to grab the ball with his arms over his head. The forward on the other team also jumped up to try to head the ball; his knee hit forcefully into the goalkeeper's abdomen, and the goalkeeper fell to the ground in pain. The referee stopped the game and the athletic training student and head athletic trainer ran onto the field to assess the goalkeeper.

The goalkeeper was in a great deal of pain and was lying on his side with his knees held near his chest. He vomited once and did not want to move or allow anyone to touch his abdomen. After a few minutes, the athletic trainers were able to calm him down, and the head athletic trainer palpated his abdomen. It was very rigid and tender, and he still did not want to move or stand up to be moved off the field. Because the school was so rural, an ambulance could take 15 to 20 minutes to arrive, but there was a small hospital on campus. The head athletic trainer suggested that she drive her car onto the field, place the goalkeeper in the backseat, and drive him directly to the hospital emergency room on campus, and the athletic training student agreed. The head athletic trainer took the goalkeeper to the hospital, and the student athletic trainer remained at the soccer field for the remainder of the game.

Discussion Questions

1. What is your differential diagnosis? How would you confirm and/or rule out each condition you suspect?

2. Do you feel that having the student transport the athlete to the hospital was the correct course of action? Why or why not? If not, how do you feel the situation should have been managed?

3. What types of protection could the goalkeeper have worn to prevent this injury? How much does each option cost? Are these options commonly used? Why or why not?

Resolution

The head athletic trainer was able to assist the goalkeeper into the emergency department in a wheelchair and have him evaluated by the medical staff within 2 minutes. The hospital staff ran several tests on the goalkeeper but could not determine his diagnosis. About 5 hours later, they considered sending him home to rest but then decided to keep him at the hospital overnight for observation. In the morning, the goalkeeper was still in considerable pain, so the physicians performed exploratory surgery in his abdomen to look for damage. His small intestine had been ruptured in the collision, but they were able to repair it. The surgery resulted in a 10-inch abdominal incision.

Historically, this injury has a high mortality rate and the hospital on campus did not have a CT scan unit or a magnetic resonance imaging unit. They saved the goalkeeper's life, but he remained in the hospital for about 1 month and was not able to return to full soccer competition for a full year.

Additional Resolution

If the student athletic trainer had this to do over again, she would do several things differently:
- Call and wait for an ambulance to transport the goalkeeper
- Have the goalkeeper transported to a better-equipped hospital with better imaging services, such as a CT scanner
- Travel with the goalkeeper to the hospital to help oversee his care and better communicate with his parents, who lived in Ireland (international student)
- Encourage the goalkeepers to wear equipment that protects their abdominal area

Notes:_____

_____

_____

_____

_____

_____

SCENARIO 10: POLE VAULTING INCIDENT

At a home high school regional level track and field meet, a senior male athlete was pole vaulting. As he was attempting to break a school record of 13'6", he heard his pole crack on his second pass. He checked his pole and found a defect, so he retrieved another standard pole vaulting pole from the locker room. He practiced a few pseudo vaults, checking the flex of this new pole. On his first pass using the new pole, he sprinted down the runway and placed the pole perfectly in the vault box. He propelled 13'6" up and cleared the cross bar but did not have the momentum needed to land in the padded landing area. He quickly descended head first, and the left side of his head struck the edge of the steel vault box. His left shoulder went into the base of the vault box, and his body was in a side lying position, halfway in the vault box and halfway out. He lay motionless and unconscious. His body was surrounded by the foam mats, which made the initial assessment/evaluation difficult due to the lack of room to access this patient.

Personnel: One athletic trainer, who had 3 years of hands-on experience, and 2 high school senior students, who had volunteered as student aides during the past 2 football seasons, were present. There were also 3 track and field coaches, who had a tremendous amount of respect and confidence for/in the athletic trainer.

Being an eye witness to this catastrophic event, I knew that EMS had to be called and that our EAP would be put to the test. I shouted out to my student aide to call EMS and give them the details that he knew. Knowing a situation like this could happen anywhere at any time, it was my protocol to practice our EAP on a scheduled basis so that all involved would know what to do if/when an emergency situation arose. Thankfully, we had just had a training review on our EAP the week prior to this event. I was hopeful that all of my staff would be able to fulfill their responsibilities.

Discussion Questions

1. You assume this is a cervical spine and/or head injury; describe your hand placements for inline stabilization.

2. How do you assess a head injury when the athlete's face and upper body are in a dependent position, face down?

3. How do you communicate your EAP and perform an initial assessment when your hands are being used for inline stabilization?

Resolution

Upon further evaluation, this athlete was unconscious for a few moments but began to regain consciousness and wanted to try and stand up. He became a bit irritated that I would not allow him to move. He rolled onto his back before I could convince him to stay still. The patient was then positioned so that his head was in a declined position within the vault box, which meant that I was lying flat on the landing mats with this athlete's head in my hands, suspended in mid-air. Due to the impact site on his left temporal bone, I had to modify my hand position for inline stabilization. One hand was under the back of his head around the occiput area and the other was placed on the right side of his head by his right ear. Once my hands were placed on this patient's head area holding stabilization, I could do no further hands-on assessment myself. I called into action my student aide to assess his pulse. I was able to visualize/observe signs and symptoms as I watched, listened, and spoke with this athlete. At this point, the patient was conscious, alert, and somewhat oriented. I maintained inline stabilization as I was calling out orders to double check that the gate was open for the EMS to enter. Now, the waiting game occurred. What seemed like 30 minutes was actually 4 minutes. The EMS crew arrived, and the patient was evaluated further, packaged, and transported to the landing zone to be life-flighted to the nearest Level I trauma unit. Final diagnosis included a concussion, fracture of the left temporal bone, rupture of the middle meningeal artery, and epidural and subdural hematomas. After 1 month of hospitalization and 2 months of recovery, this student graduated from high school, went on to college, and graduated with a degree in engineering.

Additional Resolution

Reflecting back on this incident and our EAP, the only item that was not covered in the EAP was a location for the landing zone. Fortunately, this event happened at our home school and our EMS was familiar with the layout of the land, so they were able to designate the landing zone.

Notes:_____

_____

_____

_____

_____

SCENARIO 11: BEING IN UNFAMILIAR TERRITORY AND DEALING WITH MULTIPLE INJURIES

Toward the end of the fourth quarter of an away high school football game, your senior star running back was coming around the end on the far side of the field and got hit low by a linebacker, who was blocked into him, and also got hit high by the cornerback coming up to make the tackle. There was nothing illegal about the hits.

As the athletic trainer, you knew immediately that your running back had suffered a severe injury, even from where you were standing. You knew you were supposed to wait until the game officials summoned you onto the field. You were not familiar with the local EMS crew. The host athletic trainer introduced himself to you prior to the beginning of the game with no other information.

Even though you were not summoned by the official to go onto the field, you began to make your way to your athlete because, even from a distance, it was clear that he has suffered a significant injury. Once you reached your athlete, you immediately saw that his left knee had been dislocated. His lower leg was at a 90-degree angle, laterally from the midline of his body. You immediately summoned the EMS crew, and they slowly walked to you from the other end zone. The host athletic trainer was still on his sideline, and no physician was available.

To add to the situation, the father of your athlete witnessed this all from the stands. In making his way to the field, he jumped over the fence, not realizing there was an 8-foot drop from the bleachers. He landed on the ground over by the fence and was unable to walk.

Discussion Questions

1. What should your first concern be in this situation?

2. How do you get him into the ambulance? Remember that his lower leg is out to the left at a 90-degree angle.

3. Do you respond to the father's needs? If so, how?

Resolution

The first priority had to be the athlete. I did not wait for the officials to summon me onto the field. I got halfway across the field and knew I would need additional help, including EMS, and began calling for their assistance. Whenever a knee dislocation is suspected, neurovascular assessment should immediately become the focus of the evaluation. It is important to immediately assess and compare the posterior tibial and dorsal pedal pulses if possible. If there are distal pulses, there is a bit more time to deal with the injury. If there is no distal pulse, this would then become a true medical emergency to save the lower leg. Fortunately, in this situation, we found distal pulses. An assistant coach was sent to the slow-walking EMS crew to get them to bring their ambulance and equipment onto the field as soon as possible. Once they understood the gravity of the situation, they responded accordingly, as did the host athletic trainer. My next priority was to stabilize the injury and ready the athlete for transport.

Packaging the athlete for transport presented a problem because of the way the lower leg was positioned. We needed to position the athlete on his right side while still maintaining the integrity of the distal pulses and the position of the leg to get him through the ambulance door.

Once the athlete was in the ambulance and stabilized, I felt comfortable enough to deal with the father's injury. Upon examination, I found the father in very little pain but with a large mass in the posterior of his right lower leg. He was unable to plantarflex his foot. The father appeared to have completely ruptured his Achilles tendon. I fit him with a set of crutches, wrapped an ice bag on his leg, and put him in the passenger seat of the ambulance to be transported with his son.

I notified our team physician, who then notified the hospital emergency room about the situation. A surgical reduction of the knee was performed that evening. A follow-up surgery was needed to repair the anterior and posterior cruciate ligaments, the medial collateral ligament, and a lateral meniscal tear.

The father's injury also needed to be surgically repaired. Both patients recovered fully from their injuries after extensive rehabilitation.

Notes:
_____
_____
_____
_____
_____
_____

SCENARIO 12: SOCCER GOALIE COLLISION WITH FIELD PLAYERS

An athletic trainer was covering a home soccer game. During the game, the goalie collided with 2 field players while attempting to scoop up the ball. At the point of collision, the goalie sustained a blow to his head and chest and was knocked unconscious. As the athletic trainer approached the scene, it was noted that the 2 field players were on the ground—one was lying on the ground clutching his knee and the other was sitting up and looking dazed. The goalie was in an abnormal body posture with his arms and legs held straight out, his toes pointed downward, and his head and neck arched backward. The muscles were tightened and rigid.

Through initial evaluation, the athletic trainer determined that the goalie was unconscious. He was breathing and occasionally made a grunting sound. The athletic facility's EAP was activated, and EMS was called.

Discussion Questions

1. What type of posturing is the athlete exhibiting? What does this posture suggest?

2. Did the athletic trainer make the correct decision in which athlete he treated first? What care should be given until EMS arrive?

3. What is the significance of combativeness in an athlete with a head injury?

Resolution

The athletic trainer maintained an open airway and monitored vitals while the head coach stayed alongside the athlete speaking calmly and directly to the athlete. The athlete was visibly responding to the coach's voice, and the coach was not giving any instructions, just comforting words.

The EMS unit was met and escorted to the field by an assistant coach. The athlete was back boarded without issue; however, as vitals were being taken in the ambulance, the athlete became combative and had to be restrained. The athlete was transported by ambulance to the nearest trauma center. An assistant coach accompanied the athlete to the hospital with the athlete's emergency contact and insurance information. Parents and administrators were notified of the event.

Notes:_____

_____

_____

_____

_____

_____

SCENARIO 13: BILATERAL PATELLAR TENDON RUPTURE

During a football game, an opponent's quarterback fumbled the ball and a defensive end scooped it up and started to run around the quarterback. In an instant reaction to tackle the defensive end with the ball, the quarterback reached out with arms level and horse collared the defensive end. In doing so, the defensive end was swept off his feet and came down on both knees but tried to maintain his feet under him. As the tackled defensive end lay on the turf, the athletic trainer ran out to assess the player. Upon arrival, the athletic trainer asked where the injury was located and the player said both knees. Concerned about several injuries that could have occurred, but evaluating the right patella and then moving to the left patella, the athletic trainer and team orthopedic surgeon determined that the player had sustained bilateral patellar tendon ruptures. An ambulance was in attendance, and a second athletic trainer summoned them to report with an ambulance gurney.

Discussion Questions

1. How would you assess these injuries?

2. How would you immobilize these injuries?

3. Who would be in charge of the scene?

4. How would you initiate your EAP if this occurred at practice rather than during a game?

Resolution

Due to the bilateral patellar tendon ruptures, the athletic trainer obtained 2 straight-leg knee immobilizers so each knee could be immobilized. With the gurney alongside the player, he was lifted by the orthopedic surgeon, 2 athletic trainers, and 2 paramedics. With the assistance of the ambulance gurney, the player was extricated from the field to the ambulance and then to the hospital emergency room. The following day, the player underwent bilateral patellar tendon repairs.

*Notes:*_____

_____

_____

_____

_____

_____

SCENARIO 14: EMERGENCY ABDOMINAL INJURY

A 20-year-old male intercollegiate football player presented to the athletic training room on Sunday afternoon of Memorial Day weekend with abdominal pain, nausea, and vomiting. He stated that approximately 24 hours before, he was jet skiing with friends at a local lake. He was riding with a friend on a jet ski at approximately 40 miles per hour when they attempted a sharp turn and were both thrown from the jet ski. He was struck in the abdomen by the handlebar.

The athlete appeared pale and diaphoretic. He stated that his abdominal pain had progressively worsened over the past 24 hours. He stated his pain was 9/10 on the pain scale. Of his vital signs, his pulse was 125 beats per minute, blood pressure was 102/64, and oxygen saturation was 94%. He was afebrile, and his respirations were shallow, with a rate of 22 breaths per minute. Breath sounds were clear to auscultation. Deep breathing was painful over his right side. His abdomen had an abrasion and ecchymosis over the right upper abdominal quadrant. He stated that he had urinated, that it was not painful, and that his urine appeared normal in color. He was not tender to flank palpation; however, his abdominal quadrant evaluation was markedly positive, with muscle guarding and pain, particularly over the upper right abdominal quadrant with a positive rebound sign. He had pain with palpation over the lower right ribs and had a positive rib cage compression sign without crepitus.

He stated that he had applied ice and taken both over-the-counter (OTC) anti-inflammatory medicine and acetaminophen; however, nothing helped to relieve his pain. He had no known allergies and was taking no other OTC medications, prescription medications, or supplements. His medical history was unremarkable. His last oral intake was approximately 3 hours prior; he had attempted to drink an electrolyte drink but became extremely nauseous and vomited shortly after ingestion.

Discussion Questions

1. How would you expect vital signs to trend following an acute abdominal injury?

2. Would you expect the athlete to experience any referred pain from an abdominal injury? If so, where would it possibly refer to and what sites might be indicative of injury to what structures?

3. At the time of initial evaluation (prior to emergency referral), the athlete requested to drink water. Is this appropriate? If not, why would it not be appropriate with these circumstances?

Resolution

The athlete was transported to the hospital emergency department for evaluation with a differential diagnosis of liver injury vs rib fracture vs abdominal wall contusion. His parents, head team physician, and sport coach were notified. X-rays were negative for rib fractures; however, CT scan was positive for a liver laceration. The athlete was admitted to the hospital with consults obtained by a trauma surgeon and a general surgeon, but surgery was not indicated. The athlete remained in the hospital for 3 days for monitoring and pain control. Upon discharge, the athlete was followed by the head team physician and athletic trainer. Consults and literature review were performed to determine the best treatment course. The athlete ultimately returned to football activities 4 months following injury, wearing a custom protective pad over the upper right abdominal quadrant, and completed the season without incident.

Although rare, abdominal injuries in sports can be life threatening. They require prompt evaluation and monitoring. Participation in contact/collision sports places the athlete at significant risk for reinjury. An appropriate amount of time must be allowed for healing, and protective padding should be considered with return to athletic activity.

*Notes:*_____

_____

_____

_____

_____

_____

SCENARIO 15: CERVICAL SPINE INJURY

A 21-year-old male intercollegiate football player (defensive back/kick returner; 6'0", 180 lbs) was returning a kickoff in a football game. He received the ball deep in the end zone and was tackled at the 26 yard line. Having traveled approximately 35 yards, he was at full speed at the time of the tackle. The tackler (linebacker, 6'4", 235 lbs) on the opposing team had traveled approximately 35 yards at the time of the tackle. As he was unblocked during the play, he was also traveling at full speed. The kick returner dropped his head just prior to contact, and a significant helmet-to-helmet blow occurred. The tackler was concussed on the play and required evaluation and assistance in removal from the field. The kick returner immediately jumped up following the tackle and ran to the sideline with no complaints or appearance of injury.

As the offense had the ball, the kick returner went to the defensive bench to rest. After a 10-play drive, the offense faced fourth down and elected to punt. As the defense gathered up to prepare to return to the field, the kick returner/defensive back approached the athletic trainer on the sideline and stated that there was something wrong with his neck. The athlete had palpable cervical paraspinal muscle spasm and marked cervical ROM deficits in all movement planes. The athlete was removed from activity and the coaches were notified.

The athlete was evaluated further on the sideline by the athletic trainer and team physicians. He had spinal column pain with palpation from C3 to C7, with no crepitus or deformity noted. He was neurovascularly intact with normal upper and lower extremity sensation, strength, and reflexes. He had no radicular pain. The athlete had removed his football helmet prior to reporting injury to the athletic trainer. His shoulder pads were carefully removed to avoid cervical movement, and, upon removal, a rigid cervical collar was applied. He was transported to the hospital for evaluation and the team neurosurgery consultant was notified, who met the athlete and athletic trainer at the emergency department. There was no change in his cervical examination at the emergency department. Vital signs were normal. X-rays revealed a C4-C5 fracture/subluxation. The athlete was secured to a spine board and additional studies were performed with CT scan and magnetic resonance imaging. The neurosurgeon applied Gardner-Wells tongs and traction to stabilize the spine prior to surgery.

The athlete's parents lived out of state and were not in attendance at the game. They were notified by telephone of their child's injury and the need for surgery to stabilize his cervical spine. Arrangements were made to fly the parents in, and a medical staff member and chaplain met them at the airport to transport them to hospital.

Discussion Questions

1. What is the most common mechanism of injury for a cervical spine fracture/dislocation?

2. With this athlete, concomitant head and neck injuries must be ruled out with the mechanism of injury. How does the suspected cervical spine injury impact concussion evaluation?

3. This scenario reinforces the need to have a crisis management plan. Which individuals and what actions would be indicated with a crisis management plan at your institution if one of your athletes sustained such an injury?

Resolution

The neurosurgeon performed a C4-C5 open reduction internal fixation and fusion using a bone graft from the pelvis. The athlete had an unremarkable postoperative course. He made a full recovery; however, he was medically disqualified from further football participation.

Sports health care providers in contact/collision sports are aware of the potential for cervical spine injuries; however, not all injuries present the same way. Regardless of presentation, health care providers must always be aware of the potential for spine injury with an axial load mechanism.

*Notes:*_____

_____

_____

_____

_____

_____

SCENARIO 16: RUPTURED SPLEEN IN MEN'S LACROSSE PLAYER

During the first practice of the year for the men's lacrosse team, a midfielder was checked and fell on the butt end of his lacrosse stick (cross). The cross caught him just below the left rib cage. He immediately went down and felt severe pain in that area. He walked to the sideline and was evaluated by the one of his teammates, who was a lifeguard, and knew the situation was serious.

The athletic trainer had been detained in the athletic training room and was heading to practice when he was summoned by telephone. One of the coaches had activated the EMS system.

Upon initial evaluation from the athletic trainer, the athlete was tender upon palpation over the left quadrant and he was beginning to show signs of going into shock. He was pale and was wavering in and out of consciousness. He was then placed supine on the ground, with his legs elevated about 6" off the ground. It was late January, and the athletic trainer tried to maintain normal body temperature.

The EMS arrived and transported him to the local hospital. He was evaluated in the emergency department, where it was determined that he had ruptured his spleen. The time of initial on-field evaluation to his arrival at the operating room was approximately 2.5 hours.

Discussion Questions

1. How would you initially handle this situation upon arrival to the scene?

2. What signs and symptoms would lead you to be concerned if this were a life-threatening injury?

3. If the EMS had not been contacted, how would you initiate your EAP?

Resolution

The athlete underwent a successful splenectomy and was hospitalized for 10 days. He had a full recovery and returned to lacrosse the following year.

Additional Resolution

The athletic trainer had 2 previous football players who sustained splenic injuries. These 2 did not need surgery but were hospitalized for observation. This scenario presented with an obvious and significant internal injury. The coach, teammates, and athletic trainer worked together and activated the EMS system appropriately for a successful outcome of a life-threatening situation.

Notes:_____

_____

_____

_____

_____

_____

Scenario 17: Posterior Wall Myocardial Infarction of a Football Player

A senior defensive lineman was brought to the athletic trainer by his teammates. He was showing signs of dehydration: profuse sweating, vomiting, and lethargy. It was during the acclimatization phase of practice as they were only wearing helmets.

The teammates also stated that the individual was up most of the night vomiting and had several bouts of diarrhea. He refused to see the athletic trainer, but teammates forced him to.

He was sent to the showers with a teammate and then sent to the athletic training room to remain under observation by the assistant athletic trainer. She then called and it was thought he should be seen at student health. She drove him to student health, but they were too busy to see him, so she then took him to the emergency department of the local hospital 1.5 miles away. She dropped him off and returned to the office.

Discussion Questions

1. Should a member of the school's staff stay with an athlete who has been taken to the hospital?

2. What are the signs and symptoms of a myocardial infarction (MI)? How commonly does this occur in young athletes? Did this athlete display any of the signs and symptoms?

3. What is the initial treatment for an MI?

Resolution

Upon the completion of football practice, I went to see the athlete at the emergency department. While in the room with the player, he told me that he was having a heart attack. Follow-up with a cardiologist revealed a posterior wall MI. He was admitted to the hospital for 4 days and then returned to school. He underwent a complete course of cardiac rehabilitation and was able to return to football as a student coach. He never returned to competitive football.

Additional Resolution

This situation was a team effort of the teammates and athletic training staff. No one knew the severity of the situation at the time, but if the athlete had forced the issue and returned to practice, the result could have been catastrophic. The only possible change in the scenario would have been to activate EMS. Campus safety was not available for transport as students were moving in for the fall semester.

Notes:_____

_____
_____
_____
_____
_____

SCENARIO 18: ATHLETE WITH
POST-EXERTIONAL CHEST DISCOMFORT

An athlete reported mild centralized chest discomfort post-workout. The workout included weight lifting followed by multiple sprints. He had an approximately 2-week history of upper respiratory infection symptoms, including cough. Current symptoms included retrosternal discomfort. No shortness of breath, lightheadedness, or radiating pain was reported. The athlete denied use of any OTC or prescription medicine or supplements and did not smoke.

The athlete had a history of hypertension, and his family history included the death of his father before the age of 50 years due to unknown causes. The athlete's vitals were stable and he reported no heart racing or irregular heart rate or rhythm. The team physician was consulted by telephone. Watchful waiting was recommended. The athlete was given instructions on what to look for with worsening symptoms.

Approximately 3 hours later, the athlete called the athletic trainer and stated that he had developed left-sided back pain. He continued to deny shortness of breath, dizziness, and lightheadedness. He complained of mild retrosternal pain. The team physician was contacted again and recommended that the athlete report to the emergency department for further evaluation.

Discussion Questions

1. What are the differential diagnoses with the signs/symptoms described in this scenario?

2. What are the worsening symptoms an athlete should be instructed to look for in this scenario?

3. Based on the scenario, and without input from a physician, would you have referred this athlete for an emergency department evaluation or would you let him return to normal workouts?

Resolution

After presenting to the hospital, the athlete underwent electrocardiogram, laboratory tests, and a cardiac catheterization. He had a clot at the left anterior descending coronary artery during the cardiac catheterization. He underwent 2 separate procedures to remove the clot. Additional testing revealed 5 predisposing clotting risk factors. After recovery and rehabilitation of approximately 18 months, the athlete was eventually cleared for a return to football. He played for 2 years with no further cardiac issues and led the team in number of snaps his senior year. He was on beta-blockers, which led to some adjustments in his cardiovascular training, but otherwise had no restrictions.

Additional Resolution

Additional screening tools could have been used during preseason physicals that could have identified any of the risk factors that were later identified after the MI.

Notes:_____

_____

_____

_____

_____

_____

SCENARIO 19: HIP DISLOCATION IN A HIGH SCHOOL FOOTBALL GAME

Friday night in Western Pennsylvania means high school football, and the largest schools have several thousand people in attendance. My ambulance service covers 2 high schools for varsity football, and for the past 15 years, I have worked the games at the largest school. My background as a paramedic and athletic trainer has given me a unique perspective when working these games, and the relationship between the school's athletic trainer and my EMS agency has been excellent. When working these games, I always try to make contact with the visiting athletic trainer and team physician to advise them of my location and offer to help in any way possible. I always mention my background as an athletic trainer and nurse anesthetist to assure them of my full cooperation for any injury situation.

One Friday night, the visiting athletic trainer informed me that his team orthopedic surgeon was late but would arrive shortly. During the fourth quarter, the visiting linebacker made a tackle while also being blocked, and he went down hard. He was supine on the field with his left hip flexed at 90 degrees while his knee was also flexed to 90 degrees, and the entire leg was externally rotated. He was at the opposite end of the field, but it was clear from my vantage that his hip was dislocated. I immediately told my partner to grab the stretcher, and I started running down the sidelines to the player before the play had ended.

The visiting athletic trainer and orthopedic surgeon also responded immediately, and as I approached, I could see the surgeon working to reduce the dislocation immediately. He was successful in relocating the joint, but the player was in considerable pain. My crew and I made contact with the visiting staff and we made plans for extrication and transport of the player. At this time, the home athletic trainer and orthopedic surgeon also arrived on the field and offered their assistance.

We immobilized the left leg by strapping it to the right leg to prevent the player from flexing the hip. Then, the home orthopedic surgeon demanded that we transport the player to the nearest trauma center (where he was chief of orthopedics) and that I call for trauma team activation. Because the trauma center was the closest hospital, I was going to take the player there anyway, and because the hip was relocated, I knew he did not need a trauma team. The orthopedic surgeon had an ego bigger than the moon, and he demanded that I activate the trauma team prior to transport. The visiting team staff agreed to transport to the closest facility, and the player's mother had come onto the field and also agreed with the transport. I decided that arguing with the home physician was pointless, so I ignored him.

We moved the player onto the stretcher and took him to the ambulance. In the process, we called dispatch and requested a second unit from our service to come to the stadium to take our place for the remainder of the game. Once we were in the ambulance, we started transport, with the mother riding up front. Oxygen was applied, vital signs obtained, and a large bore intravenous (IV) bag was initiated. After a 500-cc fluid bolus, I administered fentanyl 100 mcg for pain control because the athlete rated his pain at 10/10.

En route to the hospital, I called the emergency department and spoke with the attending physician. I gave him a report on the player's condition and also advised him of the demand for trauma team activation. The emergency department physician told me the home surgeon had already called him with the trauma team request, but he was waiting for my report. Upon arrival at the hospital, the player was in no pain and was singing his favorite song. In the emergency department, we were met by the attending physician and a senior orthopedic resident, who did a quick evaluation in the hallway and then directed us to a minor treatment room. The player was kept overnight for observation and discharged the next day for follow-up with the home orthopedic surgeon.

Discussion Questions

1. What are the short- and long-term advantages of rapid reduction of a dislocation on the field?

2. How would you handle the request from a home physician if it conflicted with your own evaluation?

3. What would you do to prevent a recurrence of this conflict?

Resolution

The player was lost to follow-up, and the home orthopedic surgeon did not register a complaint with my service. I advised management of the incident with a special report on my trip sheet. I also talked with the visiting orthopedic surgeon after the game and advised him of the patient's condition and my interventions. He expressed his gratitude and indicated he had no respect for the home surgeon. I also apologized for not making contact with him prior to the game; if I had been able to do so, I could have started the IV on the field and sedated the player for the reduction. He laughed and said that would have made it easier, but it never occurred to him that such services were available.

Additional Resolution

Nothing further could have been done for this situation, but future conflicts were sure to occur unless we could come to an arrangement with the home orthopedic surgeon. We had previous conflicts with this individual and, fortunately, he decided to send a resident to cover the games after this event.

Notes:_____

_____

_____

_____

_____

_____

SCENARIO 20: HELICOPTER TRANSPORT OF A FOOTBALL PLAYER WITH A HEAD INJURY

During a high school varsity football game between 2 large high schools, the home quarterback was tackled hard and struck his head on the turf violently. He did not get up, and the school's medical staff quickly responded. The player had an altered level of consciousness and reported cervical pain but was disoriented. The staff consisted of an athletic trainer, an orthopedic resident, and a family practice physician. The athletic trainer and the resident were contracted from a sports medicine clinic, while the family practice physician was employed by the school district as the official school doctor. After evaluating the player, they determined that it was necessary to immobilize him on a spine board, and EMS was summoned onto the field. The paramedics and the staff had a good relationship and were working to immobilize the player while the athletic trainer removed the facemask. Suddenly, the family practice physician informed the paramedics that they should call a helicopter to transport the player to a trauma center.

The paramedics were hesitant to call the helicopter because the trauma center was only 15 minutes away by ground and, although the player's injuries were serious, they did not arise to the level of helicopter transport. The athletic trainer and the orthopedic resident agreed with the paramedics, and an argument ensued. The family practice physician indicated that because he was the only school employee among the group, his request was paramount and again demanded for a helicopter. The paramedics relented and called dispatch for air evacuation of the player. Because this was a congested suburban area, the closest landing zone was 5 miles away, so the crew asked for the helicopter to land on the field.

This area has a plethora of medical helicopters, and when the request was made, one happened to be in the area returning from a flight. The helicopter was overhead in less than 3 minutes, and after the pilot surveyed the field, he told the paramedics he would land on the field only after the stands were evacuated of all spectators. Because there were approximately 5000 people in attendance, it took longer than 45 minutes for the evacuation to occur.

The helicopter landed on the field, and the player was transported to a trauma center. The delay for evacuation meant it took longer than 1 hour from the time of injury until the player arrived at the trauma center.

Discussion Questions

1. Explain the golden hour for trauma patients.

2. Does the employment status of the sports medicine staff make a difference when there is a disagreement over injury management?

3. Does your EAP make provisions for helicopter transport?

Resolution

The player spent several days in the hospital and was discharged with the diagnosis of a closed head injury. There was no cervical spine trauma. He was cleared to return to play at the end of the season for a playoff game, but his parents were unhappy with the entire event and refused to let him play.

Additional Resolution

The paramedics could have called their command physician and explained the situation. The command physician, who was an attending emergency doctor at the local hospital, would have then explained to the family practice physician the implications of helicopter transport and would have refused to authorize such transport. The EAP must take into account all possible scenarios no matter how remote.

Notes:_____

_____

_____

_____

_____

_____

SCENARIO 21: POST-PRACTICE IN A HURRY

A 6'5", 17-year-old high school basketball player was running out of the gymnasium after practice. When he reached the door to exit the building, he placed his left hand on the bar to push the door open and his right hand (dominant hand) on the window for additional force and continued to run through the door. The window was lined with chicken wire to reinforce the glass. Given the angle and force of the push with his right arm, his hand went through the glass and received multiple large lacerations from the glass and the chicken wire.

As the patient did not immediately recognize that he was injured, he continued to exit the door while his arm was stuck in the window. When he realized what had happened, he screamed and his coach ran to him. The coach instructed him to remove his hand from the glass and walk the approximate 40 yards to the athletic training facility. The athletic trainer heard the commotion, and when she looked into the hallway, there was blood covering the floor, walls, and ceiling for approximately 15 feet from the door; the patient was waving his arm from side to side in apparent disbelief of what he was seeing. The athletic trainer retrieved gloves, gauze, and towels from the clinic and the athletic director arrived in the hallway as the athletic trainer was approaching the athlete; the athletic trainer informed the athletic director of the situation and instructed her to call 911.

The athletic trainer, who was also an army veteran, reached the patient at the same time as a wrestling coach. The wrestling coach donned gloves and placed pressure proximal to the elbow to decrease blood flow; the athletic trainer donned gloves and began removing obvious large debris that was not embedded in the skin, muscle, or bone and then applied direct pressure to the approximate 5-inch wound on the anterior forearm. The arm was then elevated to assist in decreasing blood loss as well.

Discussion Questions

1. List as many methods to control bleeding as you can.

2. When should a tourniquet be considered?

3. Why was it important for EMS to not remove the dressings applied prior to their arrival?

Resolution

The patient began to feel lightheaded and looked pale; he was then laid down and monitored for further shock signs/symptoms. As the patient was monitored, the athletic trainer began to add additional bandages and wrap roller gauze around the wounded area. She and the wrestling coach spoke to the patient to keep him calm, including pertinent questions regarding medications and history of illness.

During this time, the principal of the school and the mother of the patient arrived at the scene. The principal tried to interject her opinion and also asked the athletic trainer to provide the mother with a detailed rundown of what was happening to her son. As the mother was obviously emotionally aggravated, the athletic trainer stated she was trying to control blood loss and cover the open wound.

Approximately 10 minutes after the initial incident, EMS arrived. All details of the incident and current vital signs were relayed to the EMS personnel; EMS did not remove any of the initial dressings that had been applied to the patient. Within 6 hours, the patient was in surgery to debride the radius, ulna, and surrounding tissue of glass; reconnect the tendons of the palmaris longus, brachioradialis, flexor carpi radialis, and flexor digitorum superficialis; as well repair the median nerve, which was also severed. Postoperatively, the patient was instructed to perform physical therapy for 3 months following a short period of immobilization. Unfortunately, the patient was noncompliant in his therapy prescription and never regained full extension of his fingers or wrist. He tried to return to basketball after 8 months but was unable to attain the proper ROM to continue effectively participating in this sport.

Additional Resolution

Given that the athletic trainer had notified the athletic director to enact the EAP, following 911 notification, the athletic trainer then informed the principal and the parents. In hindsight, it would have been more beneficial for the principal to arrive on the scene but remain uninvolved to allow the care to continue without the request for additional information/description of care being provided. The noncompliance of the patient in completing the rehabilitation program is also of major concern. It would have been preferred to have the patient attend his outpatient rehabilitation sessions as well as sessions on the school campus.

Notes:_____
_____
_____
_____

SCENARIO 22: TRAUMATIC INJURY IN MINOR LEAGUE BASEBALL

During a minor league baseball game, a base runner for the home team attempted a feet-first slide into home plate. During the slide, his right leg accidentally planted and tucked under his body as his momentum carried him forward. There was an audible snap and the athlete lay supine, reaching for his lower leg. The athletic trainer rushed onto the field and immediately noticed a gross deformity of the right lower extremity. The ankle was obviously dislocated and there appeared to be a noncompound fracture of the tibia and fibula. The medical team, consisting of the home athletic trainer and strength coach, in conjunction with the visiting team athletic trainer, quickly assessed the situation and began treating the athlete.

Discussion Questions

1. How could the home athletic trainer prepare for this event ahead of time without knowing what to expect during a home game?

2. Which medical professional(s) should be involved in resolving this situation? Could nonmedical personnel be involved? How?

3. Medically speaking, what is the top priority for the athletic trainer in this situation?

Resolution

As soon as the athletic trainer assessed the situation, he used his predetermined hand signals to call for EMS response and for transportation via field cart. These signals were outlined in the EAP that the athletic trainer had established before the season began. The strength coach was instructed to get the vacuum splints from the bench and the athletic trainer attempted to calm the athlete and keep him still. The visiting athletic trainer covered the lower leg with a towel so spectators and the athlete could not see the dislocated ankle. The athletic trainer cut the laces of the shoe and checked for a dorsalis pedis pulse, which was present. He then continued to splint the lower extremity, which immobilized the ankle and knee. Meanwhile, the team president and general manager were instructed to escort the team physician from the stands to the loading area where EMS would arrive. Using a 3-person lift and carry, the athlete was placed onto the cart and was transported to the loading area where EMS could take over his care. He was evaluated by the team physician, who instructed EMS where to transport the athlete. The athletic trainer provided EMS with a list of known allergies and previous health conditions. After the athlete was transported away, the athletic trainer called the emergency department and gave them information regarding workman's compensation insurance and billing.

Notes:_____

_____

_____

_____

_____

_____

SCENARIO 23: FOREIGN DILEMMA

During a collegiate basketball tournament outside of the continental United States, a player dove for a loose ball and ended up in a seated position. An opposing player fell and landed directly on top of the seated player's head, creating an axial load to his cervical spine. The injured player's athletic trainer immediately stabilized the head while the opponent's athletic trainer began the assessment process. The injured athlete's chief complaint was that he was unable to move his upper and lower limbs. The neck was rigid upon palpation with visible spasm. The local EMS was supposed to be on site but had left the building early and needed to be summoned. Upon their arrival 30 minutes later, it was discovered that they were not equipped with a proper spine board for transport to the local emergency department. Another obstacle to overcome was the language barrier between the local EMS personnel and both of the athletic trainers. Neither athletic trainers knew the native language spoken.

Discussion Questions

1. What can be improvised to use in the place of a cervical collar when one is not available?

2. What needs to be done to make sure the injured athlete is secured properly for transport to the local emergency department?

3. What are the possible ways athletic trainers can overcome foreign language barriers in an emergency situation?

Resolution

The communication barrier was overcome as best as possible by using key terms to the EMS attendant with limited English as well as hand signals prior to the treatment and transportation of the injured athlete. This allowed open communication and input from all responders and created a team approach. A proper spine board was delivered via another emergency crew and the athlete was placed on the spine board, with the athletic trainer stabilizing the head and controlling the situation using a counting system for everyone to follow. IV bags were then utilized to stabilize the cervical spine, substituting for a proper cervical collar by securing with roller gauze to the neck and board. The athlete's head was also secured to the board with roller gauze and tape across the forehead region. Once in the ambulance with no locking mechanism available, the gurney (with spine board on top) was placed against one wall with one EMS attendant wedging himself between the opposite wall and the gurney, providing support. During the entire transport to local emergency department, the original athletic trainer stabilized the athlete's head to make sure it was secure.

*Notes:*_____

_____

_____

_____

_____

_____

SCENARIO 24: FIGHTING FOR LIFE

I was working the finish line medical tent at a large summer road race that took place in New England. A man was brought into the medical tent because he appeared disoriented and confused upon finishing the 7-mile race. He had a larger build for a runner but appeared fit overall.

Immediately upon entry to the medical tent, his rectal temperature was taken, and it read 107°F. We quickly took him to the 100-gallon ice water immersion tub on the ground. The tub was large enough to submerge his trunk, but his arms and legs were propped out of the tub, and cold water towels were rotated over his limbs.

Initially, he was compliant with the treatment. He had obvious central nervous system dysfunction; his eyes shifted between open and shut and he continued to mutter that he thought he was dying (in between requests for a beer, as well). I monitored his rectal temperature while others worked around him to circulate the water, rotate the towels, and continue to take vitals. He became more agitated as time passed, even though his temperature began to lower to around 106°F to 105°F. He yelled at the medical staff to remove the rectal probe and became combative. He stood up in the tub and began to threaten to drown himself if we did not remove the rectal probe and allow him to leave. He counted down from 3 to 1 and dunked his head under the water but surfaced quickly. He was a large and strong individual, and at this point, the larger men working the medical tent came around to restrain him while we tried to calm him by talking to him and explaining what was going on. We needed to get him back in the water so we could continue to cool him until he was a safe temperature.

Discussion Questions

1. Do you believe that restraining this patient is the best course of action? Does this place the medical providers in danger? Are there any alternatives to treating the patient at this time, and would this change your course of action?

2. What is your top priority given this athlete's current situation? What is your next step?

3. Are you able to appropriately treat this athlete if you remove the rectal thermometer to appease the patient? Do you think this would resolve the athlete's disposition?

Resolution

After a few very tense minutes, we were able to get him to lay back in the tub, but with all the metabolic heat he created while fighting against us, his body temperature remained elevated. We continued to add ice and cool his body with the water immersion. Soon, we lowered his temperature back down to 102°F and removed him from the tub onto a recovery stretcher. He had no recollection of his actions or what he had said, but he was successfully discharged later that day with no complications from his episode of exertional heat stroke.

*Notes:*_____

_____

_____

_____

_____

SCENARIO 25: TRAUMATIC BRAIN INJURY IN A TRACK AND FIELD ATHLETE

At a large collegiate track and field meet, a 19-year-old male hammer thrower was warming up prior to the start of the official warm-up. No track meet official was present in the area. The athlete threw his hammer and was going out to retrieve it. He was walking just outside the boundary facing away from the platform. He was wearing a hooded sweatshirt. The next athlete noted the athlete was outside the boundary and made his warm-up throw. During the throw, the hammer was slipping from his hand, and he let go. The errant throw headed for the athlete. Although he and other athletes yelled, the first athlete did not react. He was struck in the posterior aspect of the head by the hammer. The athletic trainers were summoned. They arrived at the athlete's side in approximately 90 seconds and found an unconscious, nonresponsive individual. He had a pulse and had adequate breathing. Upon palpation of the head, they could feel a depressed skull where the hammer had hit. His pupils were equal and reactive, although slow. During the assessment, it was noted the athlete's lips were starting to turn cyanotic, but no other obvious injuries were found. The EAP was initiated.

Discussion Questions

1. What are the implications of intubating patients with severe head injuries in the field?

2. When should oxygen and mask ventilation be performed in an unconscious patient?

3. How would you handle bleeding from a head injury?

Resolution

The EAP was initiated. Local EMS was called, and emergency equipment from the athletic training area at the track and the main athletic training room was brought to the scene. The athletic trainers immobilized the athlete and did a modified jaw thrust to open the airway. An oral pharyngeal airway was put in place, which maintained an open airway. A secondary survey was performed, and no other injuries were noted. The home school's neurosurgeon was contacted and informed of the situation. He was at the hospital and was going to meet the athlete in the emergency department. He put an operating room on standby. The EMS arrived, started an IV, immobilized the athlete on a backboard, and transported him to the hospital. He was in the operating room in less than 30 minutes from the time of the accident. He never regained consciousness and remains in a coma. His mother was trained as a care giver.

Additional Resolution

Although the outcome was tragic, the EAP worked very well in this case. All of the staff and athletic training students involved followed the plan and excellent emergency care was rendered.

Notes:_____

_____

_____

_____

_____

_____

4

Domain IV
Treatment and Rehabilitation

SCENARIO 1: CONFLICT WITH PARENT DURING PATIENT REHABILITATION

You were rehabilitating a 16-year-old football running back following his left anterior cruciate ligament reconstruction. The surgeon had provided you with the rehabilitation protocol he wanted you to follow. The patient was 3 weeks postoperative; his left knee was in a postoperative brace and he was on crutches until he was able to maintain full knee extension and demonstrate a normal gait. It was evident from his behavior that he was bored with the limited exercises he was able to do within the confines of the rehabilitation protocol. You had explained to him the healing process and why the program was limited in this early phase of healing. One day, his father accompanied him into your athletic training facility to observe his rehabilitation. Halfway through the patient's rehabilitation program, he stopped you to discuss his son's program and progression. The father let you know that he was a dentist, so he "knows all about healing," and he was concerned that you were not moving his son along quickly enough in his rehabilitation. The father pointed out that Adrian Peterson, a running back for the Minnesota Vikings, had the same procedure performed on him and was performing his offseason workouts 3 months after his injury. He reported that because his son was as exceptional as Adrian Peterson, he should be doing more aggressive exercises in his rehabilitation program.

Gorse KM, Feld F, Blanc RO, eds.
Athletic Training Case Scenarios:
Domain-Based Situations and Solutions (pp 141-170).
© 2016 Taylor & Francis Group.

Discussion Questions

1. Although the patient displayed discontent with the rehabilitation program with his behavior during his rehabilitation exercises, he never said anything about it to you. His father is now coming to you and indicating concern that he does not feel you realize the quality of athlete with which you are dealing. What should you do to satisfy both of their concerns with the program you are using?

2. How do you respond to the patient's father?

3. What could you do to make the exercises more acceptable to the patient but remain within the protocol restrictions?

Resolution

It is important to display confidence and calmness when dealing with an irate parent. Reacting with concern and respect is appropriate, regardless of how the individual reacts to you. You should express gratitude for the father's knowledge of healing and inform him that you do not often encounter parents with this information, so you are grateful. You should also point out that no 2 athletes should be compared to each other, for each person is different. Mr. Peterson's return to sports participation was certainly unique and rapid, but not everyone should expect the same result within the same time frame.

You should indicate that you are sorry that the father and son are displeased with the rehabilitation progression and let them know that you will try to explain to them why this is the case. You are required to follow the physician's orders, and the patient's physician provided you with a specific protocol he wanted you to follow for this patient's rehabilitation program. You are governed by the boundaries of the law and have no choice but to abide by the guidelines of this program. If they are dissatisfied with the program, they must discuss it with the surgeon; you are bound to abide by whatever instructions the physician provides you.

Although exercises are limited in the early phases of rehabilitation, changing some of the exercises and mixing them up may resolve some of the patient's complaints. For example, using manual resistance rather than weights may be more exciting for him.

Notes:_____

_____

_____

_____

_____

_____

SCENARIO 2: QUESTION OF APPROPRIATE PROCEDURE

Your intercollegiate softball center fielder suffered a Grade III sprain of the right anterior talofibular ligament and a Grade II sprain of the calcaneofibular ligament in June during the last game of the season. She hit a ball into left field and was running to second base. She suffered the injury when her foot stuck on the base and her body kept moving. The ankle and foot were placed in a walking boot for 6 weeks. She went home for the summer before the boot was removed. In August, she reported that she did not do any rehabilitation for the injury while she was gone. You started working with her to rehabilitate the ankle. You noticed yesterday, the first day you saw her, that her foot, ankle, and leg had a lot of swelling; she explained that that was how it had been since the boot was removed. You measured the calf and ankle and saw that they were both 1" larger than the left side. You used modalities, elevation, and a compression stocking to reduce the swelling. When yesterday's treatment was completed, you were pleased to see that the edema was reduced by 5/8". You instructed her to keep the limb elevated overnight and move the ankle to pump the fluid into the lymph system. Today, you saw that the swelling had returned despite the fact that she told you she followed your instructions. You called the orthopedic physician to let him know about the swelling, but he told you that it was normal and that you should continue with her rehabilitation program.

Discussion Questions

1. What do you suspect is the reason for her persistent swelling? What tests could help you determine if this is the case?

2. If the test you perform is positive, will you do as the orthopedic physician has instructed and continue with her rehabilitation?

3. What is the best way to resolve this issue?

Resolution

Swelling like this should raise a red flag, especially following surgery or a time of immobilization. The clinician should think that this may be deep vein thrombosis. The test to use to rule this condition out is the Homans sign.

If the test is positive, the patient needs to have a Doppler test to confirm the diagnosis. However, the Doppler test must be ordered by a physician. You should refrain from exercises until deep vein thrombosis has been ruled out.

If the orthopedic physician is someone you have a good relationship with and listens to you, you may want to contact him again and explain the results of your test and your concerns. If this is not possible, then the team's general practitioner or the patient's primary care physician should be contacted. It is likely that the physician will want the patient to have a Doppler performed as soon as possible.

Notes:_____

_____

_____

_____

_____

SCENARIO 3: ATHLETE WITH PSYCHOLOGICAL ISSUES RESULTING FROM A CONCUSSION

The head coach of the football team at a Division III college tells you, the athletic trainer, about the great transfer running back that they have coming in for the upcoming season. The coach mentioned that he was a Division I transfer and was 5'11" and 235 lbs. He was a national powerlifting champion in high school and purportedly ran a 4.5-second 40-yard dash.

He arrived for the first day of fall camp looking even more impressive physically than the previous descriptions. He was in phenomenal physical condition and was eager to begin practice. The first 3 practices of the season were helmets only, and he performed exceptionally well; he was fast, smooth, and strong. All of the coaches and staff could not wait to get him in pads and see what he looked like when the hitting began.

On the fourth day of camp, the players come out in full pads, and everyone looks forward to the sounds of pads popping and full-contact football. As the running backs completed their individual drills, the transfer running back looked as impressive as ever. Finally, the time had come for the hitting drills, and the coaches lined up the running backs across from the defensive players. It was a full-contact drill and the runners were to be tackled by the defensive players. The transfer running back was first in line and took off toward the defense on the whistle. Just as he was about make contact, he fumbled the ball and fell on the ground to recover. The coaches did not think anything of it and told him to jump back in line. On his second turn, he took off at the whistle and stumbled and fell just as he was about to make contact with the defense. Again, the coaches encouraged him and told him to take another repetition. This time, he began on the whistle and started chopping his feet in place and waiting for the defense player to hit him. He made no forward movement toward the defensive player at all. After this repetition, the coaches asked him about it, and he said, "I just need to get used to getting hit again."

This same scenario was repeated the following day when the running back was performing in any drill when he was going to get hit by a defensive player. At the end of practice, the coaches called the team together for a full-contact scrimmage. They wanted to see what the running back could do under a game-like scenario. The running back seemed excited, and the quarterback called for a hand-off to the running back on the first play. The ball was snapped and the running back took the hand-off and began toward the line of scrimmage. Just before he was to be hit by the defense, he threw the ball forward and stumbled and fell on the turf. The coaches and athletic training staff stood together to try to digest what was wrong with the running back.

Discussion Questions

1. What issues are you concerned about with the running back? What is posttraumatic stress disorder and does he show signs of it?

2. How would you go about beginning a conversation with the running back about his issues and concerns?

3. What type of interventions/referral(s) do you think would be appropriate for the running back and how would you facilitate this?

Resolution

The athletic trainer approached the running back and asked if they could talk. The running back seemed bummed out but said, "sure." After a few minutes of questioning, the running back told the athletic trainer that he had a severe concussion at his previous school and that he had not played the majority of the previous season due to the concussion. He said all of his concussion-like symptoms had resolved and that he had not experienced any symptoms in more than 6 months. Nothing that he had done over the last few days of practice had elicited any symptoms from him. In further discussion with the athletic trainer, the running back revealed that he felt like he had a mental block about getting hit and that he could not force himself to initiate contact. He had never gotten over his previous concussion.

After consultation with the coach, the athletic trainer referred him to a sports psychologist for further evaluation and counseling. He worked with the sports psychologist for several weeks as he attempted to continue noncontact practice. The psychologist had him try techniques such as mental imagery, positive self-talk, and relaxation. After many weeks of intervention, he began to make progress and eventually returned to full-contact football practice. Although he made progress, he did not progress enough during the season to play in a varsity game. Following the season, he decided to end his football career and concentrate on his studies. In conversations with the athletic trainer and coach, he said that he felt a lot better about the end of his career and that he was happy that he was able to overcome his psychological issues with the concussion.

*Notes:*_____

_____

_____

_____

_____

SCENARIO 4: FATIGUE AND IRON SUPPLEMENTATION

A female collegiate cross-country runner reported to the athletic training room with fatigue. She reported no abdominal pain, nausea, or vomiting. An athletic trainer took a medical history, including vital signs (which were normal), and determined that she was not in need of emergent care. The athletic trainer scheduled a follow-up visit with the head team physician. In the interim, the head cross-country coach decided to arrange an appointment to have this athlete receive iron infusion therapy. Prior to follow-up care with the team physician, it was determined that this athlete had received several infusions.

Discussion Questions

1. Is iron infusion therapy warranted? Why or why not?

2. Does iron infusion therapy require a prescription? Who is responsible for incurring the cost of these treatments?

3. Is iron infusion therapy considered doping? Why or why not?

Resolution

A standard protocol for this scenario would include the athletic trainer taking a thorough medical history and then referring the athlete to his or her team physician for further follow-up care. This may include laboratory tests to determine blood count, iron panel, ferritin, thyroid stimulating hormone, and free thyroxine. A consultation with a nutritionist to determine if the athlete was ingesting an adequate caloric intake and a psychologist if the athlete was suspected of having an eating disorder may be warranted as well.

Notes:_____

_____

_____

_____

_____

_____

SCENARIO 5: SQUATTING AND LOWER EXTREMITY RANGE OF MOTION

A football player reported to his athletic trainer with low back pain after squatting in the weight room. The athlete reported he was squatting below parallel and that he felt an onset of pain when returning from the deepest part of the movement. A lumbar scan examination revealed localized low lumbar pain with end range flexion and extension range of motion (ROM) testing. Neurological testing was within normal limits. As part of the examination, the athletic trainer asked the athlete to demonstrate his squatting motion while keeping his heels on the ground. During the squat, the athlete was able to bring his thighs below parallel, but just before the parallel position, his lumbar spine flexed and his hips rotated to the left. Pain was reported at the time of these compensatory movements. Further evaluation of the lower extremities was performed to determine the source of the compensatory movements. Hip and knee ROM were within normal limits. Left ankle dorsiflexion was 20 degrees, but right ankle dorsiflexion was limited at 5 degrees. The athletic trainer hypothesized that the limited right ankle dorsiflexion prevented the athlete from preforming a squat below parallel in a symmetrical manner with a neutral spine. The athletic trainer surmised that the compensatory motions required to squat below parallel produced injurious overload to the lumbar spine and the resultant pain. The strength coach wanted the athlete back in the weight room squatting as soon as possible. The athletic trainer knew he could not safely return the athlete to squatting below the parallel without addressing the ROM limitation in the right ankle.

Discussion Questions

1. If the strength coach insists on the athlete continuing to squat, what suggestions could you make to protect the athlete's back while he still has limited ankle dorsiflexion ROM?

2. What treatment techniques could you use to restore normal ankle dorsiflexion ROM if the origin of the restriction is intra- or extra-articular in nature?

3. What self-treatment techniques could you teach the athlete to him improve his ankle dorsiflexion ROM?

Resolution

The athletic trainer explained the effect of the limited ankle dorsiflexion ROM on proper squatting technique and the relationship of compensatory movements to his low back pain. The athletic trainer demonstrated the compensatory movements to the athlete by having the athlete squat in front of a mirror.

The athletic trainer met with the strength coach and explained the effect the athlete's limited right ankle dorsiflexion had on his squat form. Bringing the strength coach to the athletic training room to observe the athlete squat further clarified the compensatory movements.

The athletic trainer suggested limiting squat ROM to parallel and placing a 2-by-4 under the athlete's heels during squatting to eliminate the need for the compensatory movements. The 2-by-4 reduces the amount of ankle dorsiflexion required to squat through full range. Loads were limited to the point where squatting could be performed in a pain-free manner. Although the goal was parallel squatting, the actual range was limited to that which could be performed symmetrically with a neutral spine posture and no low back pain.

The athletic trainer further assessed the ankle to determine the source of the limited right ankle dorsiflexion ROM. Dorsiflexion ROM was limited to the same amount when tested with the knee straight or bent. This finding suggested the restricted ROM was probably due to soleus tightness or restricted talocrural joint arthrokinematic joint play. Articular glide testing of the talus in the mortise revealed that posterior glide of the talus was hypomobile. This finding suggested restricted joint arthrokinematics and possible soleus tightness were the sources of the restricted dorsiflexion. The athletic trainer addressed the limited arthrokinematic posterior glide of the talus with joint mobilization, performing Grade III-IV posterior talar glides. Mobility of the proximal and distal tibiofibular joints should be assessed due to their contribution to dorsiflexion. Any residual loss of dorsiflexion once the posterior glide was restored was addressed with myofascial release (eg, hand applied, instrumented, foam roller, roller stick) and stretching techniques directed at the soleus. Restoring the ankle dorsiflexion ROM would take several weeks.

The athletic trainer instructed the athlete in self-mobilization, self-myofascial release, and self-stretching techniques to maintain the ankle dorsiflexion ROM.

Return to below parallel squatting was only allowed when the athlete could demonstrate the ability to perform a below parallel symmetrical squat while maintaining a neutral spine position without pain.

*Notes:*_____

_____

_____

_____

SCENARIO 6: IT'S JUST A BRUISE

During football season, the basketball coach asked if you had seen one of his star players who was on the football team. He said he was hit in his bicep and was reporting not being able to straighten his arm. Not having any awareness of this problem, the player was sought out and evaluated. When he presented, he held his arm with his elbow flexed at 90 degrees, was point tender over his bicep, had very rigid muscle tone, and had ROM of approximately 30 degrees. He reported getting hit hard with a facemask in a game about 2 weeks prior but had not reported the injury. Subsequently, in practice, he got hit pretty hard every couple of days in the same spot, again never reporting the injury. Upon referral to the team orthopedist, the x-ray showed early stages of myositis ossificans.

The football coaches claimed to be unaware of the limited motion but offered little explanation to not noticing limitations in the weight room while he was performing upper body exercises. The athlete was a starter who was one of the larger skilled players and an average student who attended school for the opportunity to participate in sports.

Discussion Questions

1. What circumstances are commonly associated with the development of myositis ossificans within a bicep muscle?

2. What type of custom pad would you construct to protect this athlete from receiving a subsequent contusion to the bicep muscle that would be functional for football participation and in compliance with the National Federation of State High School Associations football rules?

3. The basketball coach is pointing fingers at the football coach, implying that he neglected to have the athlete looked at so he could keep playing. As an athletic trainer, how would you address the situation if you were brought into the athletic director's office to address these allegations?

Resolution

At the time, the team orthopedist treating the patient indicated the process had begun, and while little could be done to reverse what had already occurred, they could work to regain ROM and strength, minimize adhesions of the muscle to the newly formed bone as it matured, and protect it from future contusion. Return to participation in football was possible if these goals were met.

The athlete was restricted from contact participation in practice and was restricted from contact participation until ROM could be returned to normal limits. He was referred to formal physical therapy, where ultrasounds and ROM exercises were performed 3 days per week.

With aggressive physical therapy, ROM was re-established within a few weeks, strength was adequate, and return to football was allowed, with an extensive custom hard shell surrounding the entire bicep well hidden under the pads and jersey. The athlete was able to finish the football season, which culminated in the playoffs with a loss at the state finals. He successfully competed in the entire basketball season while wearing a protective pad and continued ROM and strengthening with close monitoring.

Additional Resolution

Failures in communication occurred between the athlete and the athletic trainer and with the coaching staff and the athlete trainer. This athlete was a powerhouse on the team, even with one nonfunctional arm. His desire to play overruled good sense to see the athletic trainer for an early evaluation. This delay in treatment and protection was quite possibly a significant factor in allowing this initial contusion to develop into myositis ossificans, causing him to miss multiple games.

Although we cannot always walk into a new situation and get the trust and support of all of the coaching staff and athletes, it should be a major objective of every athletic trainer to strive to acquire a level of trust from the earliest point possible in their career. This scenario was used in subsequent years as an example of the importance of how early recognition and treatment can help to minimize time loss, but it was an unfortunate situation for this individual.

Subsequently, the bone matured within the muscle and was very prominent on x-rays. Recommendations were made to have the growth surgically removed if he was planning to continue with collegiate-level football participation.

Notes:_____

_____

_____

_____

SCENARIO 7: MANAGEMENT OF OVERUSE INJURIES IN THE HIGH SCHOOL THROWING ATHLETE

A 16-year-old elite high school baseball pitcher presented to the athletic trainer with an elbow that had caused him pain on and off for the past year. The young athlete stated that he had accumulated more than 200 innings over his 3-year high school career. He had been examined by 4 orthopedic surgeons, who had diagnosed the injury as a low-grade strain (Grade 1) to the ulnar collateral ligament (UCL). Two of the orthopedic surgeons had recommended surgery and 2 had recommended conservative management consisting of 6 weeks of rest and rehabilitation. The literature has published numerous studies supporting a successful return to previous level of competition from surgery as well as conservative management of rest and rehabilitation.

Discussion Questions

1. What studies would you present to the athlete and his family to help them make their decision?

2. What percentages of success (return to their previous level of competition) could you present to the athlete and family to support proceeding with the surgery? Estimated time in months of return?

3. What percentages of success (return to their previous level of competition) could you present to the athlete and family to support conservative management? Estimated time in months of return?

Resolution

The player elected to undergo the UCL surgery. Most of the literature supported that 75% of players will return to their previous level of competition, leaving 25% who do not. Within the 25% who do not return, there are unforeseen complications in 5% that may result in additional procedures. The estimated time of return is 12 to 18 months. The literature also supports that there is a 25% success rate in conservative management with 6 weeks of rest and rehabilitation, followed by an interval throwing program that builds the player back into competition. The UCL reconstructive surgery was invented by Dr. Frank Jobe in 1974. Since then, the procedure has been slightly altered, most notably by Dr. Neal ElAttrache and Dr. Altchek, who altered the original technique by drilling fewer holes, creating a docking procedure, and adding an interference screw for stability and strength. All 3 techniques have high success rates. Within the past 6 years, prolotherapy has been introduced as a means of conservative management for low-grade injuries to the UCL. Platelet-rich plasma injections and stem cell injections (iliac crest proliferation) are 2 options that orthopedic surgeons have performed.

*Notes:*_____

_____

_____

_____

_____

_____

SCENARIO 8: OS TRIGONUM FRACTURE IN A COLLEGIATE BASEBALL PLAYER

A 19-year-old collegiate baseball player presented on the practice field with pain in the right ankle after sliding feet first into second base while attempting to steal. After performing an initial assessment on the field, the athletic trainer assisted the athlete, who was unable to fully bear weight, in getting to the dugout. The athlete denied any previous injury to the right ankle and described medial and lateral ankle pain and pain with plantarflexion. During the physical examination, there was moderate effusion initially but no crepitus on palpation. Special testing yielded a positive anterior drawer and a positive talar tilt laterally and medially; percussion tests were negative. Functionally, the patient continued to have pain with active and passive plantarflexion and inversion as well as passive dorsiflexion. He also demonstrated a significant antalgic gait. An initial diagnosis was made of a Grade II lateral ankle sprain. Following the application of ice, compression, and elevation, the athlete was provided with a compression wrap, placed in an Aircast Air-Stirrup ankle brace, and given crutches, with instructions to avoid weightbearing. On the day following the injury, the athlete reported to the athletic training room with a significant hemarthrosis that had expanded into the foot and toes. Cryotherapy treatment was instituted, and the athlete was instructed to continue with nonweightbearing ambulation. Over the next 2 weeks, a traditional ankle sprain protocol was utilized. The athlete's condition slowly improved, as evidenced by a decrease in ankle and foot effusion and improvements in ROM, but he was unable to fully bear weight on the ankle pain free, particularly when asked to rise onto his toes or perform any provocative cutting maneuvers.

Discussion Questions

1. Describe the signs and symptoms of an ankle injury that would trigger referral for an x-ray.

2. What type of medical procedure would be needed to correct an os trigonum fracture of the right talus?

3. Describe a rehabilitation program for an athlete recovering from an os trigonum fracture of his right talus.

Resolution

After consulting with the team physician, it was recommended that x-rays of the right ankle be obtained; upon review, it was determined that the athlete had a moderate-sized os trigonum fracture on the posterior aspect of the right talus. Surgery was quickly scheduled to resect the fracture fragment. Following surgery, the athlete was placed in a ROM walker locked in neutral for 10 days. A bone stimulator was also prescribed to facilitate healing of the fracture site. A gradual progression from partial weightbearing in the ROM walker to full unsupported weightbearing was then initiated over the next 4 weeks. Progressive ROM and strengthening exercises were incorporated simultaneously in the rehabilitation. Functional activity was initiated 6 weeks postoperatively and the athlete eventually returned to full activity 8 weeks following the initial injury.

Additional Resolution

Most importantly, I would have a lower threshold for suspecting a more significant injury in light of the significant hemarthrosis on day 2 of the injury. This should have triggered a timelier referral to the team physician and would likely have led to x-rays or a computed tomography scan being performed sooner. Os trigonum fractures are very rare and often overlooked in favor of a lateral ankle sprain.

Notes:_____

_____

_____

_____

_____

SCENARIO 9: ACHILLES TENDON RECONSTRUCTION

Following an Achilles tendon reconstruction on March 12, 2014, a postoperative splint was applied and the patient was required to be nonweightbearing. Upon returning in 2 weeks to the orthopedic surgeon, a boot walker was applied for 2 weeks with continued nonweightbearing, but the patient was instructed to remove the boot walker and perform active ankle ROM but no passive ROM. The patient returned 2 weeks later, and the surgeon instructed the patient to begin partial weightbearing while on crutches and in the boot walker and continue active ROM, but no passive ROM, out of the boot walker. Upon returning 2 weeks later (6 weeks postoperatively on April 22, 2014), the surgeon instructed the patient to begin aggressive ROM and resume weightbearing and walking slowly as tolerated. The goal for return to play was 4- to 6-month postoperative recovery.

Discussion Questions

1. What type of rehabilitation protocol is the patient doing?

2. What will be his timeline for return to sport?

3. Why is this protocol being followed for this patient?

Resolution

Due to an early motion protocol, the patient returned to full football participation in 5 months.

*Notes:*_____

_____

_____

_____

_____

_____

SCENARIO 10: SUBSCAPULAR BURSITIS IN A BASEBALL CATCHER

A 20-year-old baseball catcher who was right-hand dominant came to the training room with right posterior shoulder pain postgame. He had no history of shoulder issues. He was involved in a tagging collision at home plate at the top of the second inning, and he reported that he started to feel some stiffness for the remainder of the inning in his posterior shoulder thereafter. He continued to play in the game at his position. Initially, there was little discomfort and he was able to continue to throw and bat; however, as the game continued, he started to notice increasing discomfort in the posterior shoulder and scapular area as he continued to throw. He stayed in the game at his position and made throws back to the pitcher and second base. In addition to some more increasing sharp pain at times with the endpoint of his swing while batting, he continued with activity. He started to ensue with some degree of fatigue by the end of the game, but he was able to complete play. He was examined in the training room postgame by the athletic trainer.

Discussion Questions

1. Do you think the player should have been removed from the game considering the injury?

2. What tests would you perform between innings to further evaluate this injury?

3. Do you feel this case should have been handled more conservatively? If yes, explain.

Resolution

Gross evaluation revealed no swelling, scars, warmth, rashes, bruising, or alignment asymmetry. Active ROM was full, with some endpoint forward flexion discomfort and mild discomfort above 45 degrees of internal rotation. The acromioclavicular joint was nontender without swelling. No capsular tenderness in the glenohumeral joint was producible to palpation. Rotator cuff strength, external and internal rotation, and full can test was full. Speed's and Yergason's tests were with full strength as well. O'Brien's test was negative. Anterior slide was negative for instability. Sulcus was negative. He was palpably tender on the medial border of the right scapula, with increasing pain with scapular compression. Manual manipulation of the scapula increased pain as well. No clear rib cage tenderness throughout the costovertebral articulations or the thoracic spine was demonstrated. Cervical mobility was fully intact and there was no numbness or tingling in the upper extremity.

A magnetic resonance image (MRI) was conducted on the right shoulder with attention to the scapula and posterior thoracic wall. The MRI revealed substantial increasing edema and swelling in the interspace just anterior to the scapula posterior to the thoracic wall, consistent with subscapular bursitis. No evident edematous changes consistent with a bone contusion of the scapula or rib cage were seen. There are no fractures, and the rotator cuff was fully intact. It was more of a tendinopathy and had not shown any clear increasing edema or fluid into the subacromial or subdeltoid bursas.

The initial course of treatment was to start the player on a 10-day course of indomethacin 75 mg, 1 orally twice daily. He was shut down from any throwing activity throughout this duration but was continued with rotator cuff activation and eccentric and isometric exercises in addition to e-stimulation, ultrasound, and cryotherapy in the training room under the guidance of his athletic trainers.

His overall discomfort improved dramatically; however, he had significant pain while swinging a bat and throwing after the course of indomethacin was completed.

Musculoskeletal ultrasound–guided injection on the subacromial bursa was conducted thereafter for a more aggressive chance at analgesic control and symptom resolution.

The patient continued his athletic training room program, was re-evaluated 4 days postoperatively, and was found to have full active ROM of the right shoulder with full strength and pain.

We started to institute a 7-day interval throwing program under the guidance of his athletic trainers, which he was able to complete successfully. By day 5, he was back in the batting cages swinging pain free. He was released for full return to play 27 days postinjury.

Notes:_____

_____

_____

SCENARIO 11: PATHOKINESIOLOGY OF THE SHOULDER COMPLEX IN A THROWING ATHLETE

A freshman football quarterback reported to the athletic training facility during preseason training camp complaining of intermittent shoulder pain in his dominant right arm after repetitive bouts of throwing, which had been present for approximately 3 weeks. The pain was exacerbated with long passes that required a greater extent of arm cocking. He had been independently managing his condition with ice, over-the-counter analgesics, and minor stretching exercises but noticed no improvement; instead, the pain was worsening and negatively affecting his throwing performance. His subjective history revealed that he had suffered from a similar issue before in his senior year of high school as a pitcher during baseball season, but not to this extent and he never sought treatment. He described the pain as sharp and rated it as a 5/10 at rest that elevated to a 9/10 with activity. He recalled a vague history of a few minor shoulder injuries in high school but did not remember specific diagnoses. He had not sought medical attention for any shoulder injury since the beginning of the football summer training program. He denies any pain in his neck, elbow, or hand and reported no neurological symptoms. No obvious deformity, signs of acute edema, effusion, or ecchymosis were noted upon inspection of the affected shoulder. Static postural analysis revealed that the patient presented with slight kyphosis of the thoracic spine and that his right shoulder rested slightly inferior compared to the left. Palpation elicited point tenderness along the posterior shoulder complex, with pain produced upon palpation of the supraspinatus and infraspinatus tendons. ROM assessment yielded pain only with passive, active, and resistive (+3/5) glenohumeral external rotation when the arm was positioned in 90 degrees of abduction. Greater appreciable measures of passive and active glenohumeral external rotation were noted when the arm was abducted to 90 degrees compared to the uninvolved shoulder. In contrast, lesser appreciable measures of passive and active glenohumeral internal rotation were observed when the arm was positioned in 90 degrees of abduction when compared to the uninvolved shoulder. A scan of scapulothoracic mechanics revealed no appreciable clinical implications or bilateral differences. Evaluation of accessory joint motion for the involved shoulder exhibited hypermobility with anterior glide and hypomobility with posterior glide of the humeral head on the glenoid fossa. Special tests for subacromial impingement and labral lesions were negative. Tests of joint instability were negative; however, ironically, the anterior apprehension test provoked pain in the posterior shoulder that was alleviated with relocation of the humeral head. Upon this feedback, the athletic trainer applied a brief battery of moderate amplitude posteriorly directed joint oscillations to the shoulder and had the athlete simulate throwing mechanics immediately afterward. The athlete reported a marked decrease in pain following the oscillations. A sound neurovascular examination was deemed to be within normal limits.

Discussion Questions

1. Based on the subjective history alone, what is your clinical impression for the differential diagnosis of this musculoskeletal issue?

2. When accounting for the objective components of the physical examination, in conjunction with the patient's history, what is your clinical impression for the preliminary or provisional diagnosis of this musculoskeletal issue?

3. Based on the preliminary or provisional diagnosis, how would you manage this case? Discuss any potential relevant therapeutic treatment strategies and techniques, including the modification of strength training exercises and throwing guidelines during practice.

Resolution

The athletic trainer's clinical impression was that the athlete presented with signs and symptoms indicative of posterior internal impingement. Accordingly, the athletic trainer explained to the athlete that the hypermobility of his anterior shoulder capsule in tandem with hypomobility of the posterior capsule and surrounding tissues could have caused the humeral head to excessively glide anteriorly during the cocking phase of his overhead throwing mechanics. This results in the posterior rotator cuff tendons impinging upon the glenoid rim with abduction and extreme external rotation of the shoulder, which is a condition specific to competitive overhead throwers. A magnetic resonance arthrogram revealed no intra-articular lesions; however, the radiologist noted minor thickening of the infraspinatus and supraspinatus tendons. The athletic trainer worked with the strength and conditioning specialists to modify the athlete's resistance training routine. This consisted of excluding weighted triceps dips and replacing the barbell bench press with dumbbell floor press in his particular regimen to prevent excessive loading of the hypermobile anterior capsule. The athletic trainer also incorporated Maitland Grade III-IV joint mobilizations to address the posterior shoulder capsule hypomobility, along with Blackburn and rhythmic stabilization exercises in simulated positions of the cocking phase to improve strength and neuromuscular control, respectively. Furthermore, the athletic trainer instructed the athlete on how to independently perform the sleeper, rollover sleeper, and cross-arm stretch as a means to address stiffness of the posterior rotator cuff tendons to supplement the joint mobilization treatment for improving the glenohumeral internal rotation deficit. Pain was used as a guide in reintroducing the athlete back to activity without restrictions

*Notes:*_____

_____

_____

_____

_____

_____

SCENARIO 12: TREATMENT OF A CUMULATIVE TRAUMA DISORDER IN THE WORKPLACE

A 50-year-old female presented to your clinic for a consultation. She reported a frontal headache and pain along the occiput and the right upper trapezius. She denies radicular symptoms but stated that her symptoms had progressively worsened over the past 4 weeks. She had worked as an information technology manager for the past 5 years and did computer/desk work for 8 to 10 hours per day. She had changed workstations about 3 months previously due to a move to another building and did not recall any similar occurrence of symptoms before now.

Discussion Questions

1. How do you best determine the work-relatedness of this injury?

2. If work-related, what onsite resources could be used for addressing her work area?

3. What recommendations do you provide for the workplace?

Resolution

The patient had developed a cumulative trauma disorder, which led to trigger points along her levator scapulae, trapezius, and sternocleidomastoid muscles. Due to her recent workstation change, she had not been using an ergonomically neutral workstation, which requires a forward leaning head and outstretched, elevated arm. This was a work-related injury, and you referred her to the onsite occupational health clinic for evaluation and a workstation evaluation by the industrial hygienist. The occupational health facilitator referred her back to your clinic, and your treatment plan included mental health, trigger point therapy, postural progressive resistive exercises, and instruction in workstation microbreak exercises/stretches once per hour.

Notes:_____

_____

_____

_____

_____

_____

SCENARIO 13: TREATMENT FOR
CHRONIC LOW BACK PAIN IN A FEMALE ROWER

A 22-year-old female former Division I rower reported chronic low back pain that was unresolved via traditional therapy treatments (moist heat and electrical stimulation). Although she was otherwise fit and well conditioned, she was unable to participate in any exercise that required her to stand or sit for more than 15 minutes due to pain over her right sacroiliac joint and had severe spasms in her paraspinal musculature (L3-S1). She had a history of right shoulder anterior inferior instability that was treated previously with therapeutic exercise; she was released from outpatient physical therapy after an 8-week rehabilitation program that had been completed 6 months prior. Physical examination revealed knots throughout her paraspinal musculature, greater on the right side than the left, and point tenderness over the sacroiliac joints bilaterally. She reported pain and had limited ROM with trunk flexion and extension, as well as lateral bending and trunk rotation bilaterally. The right anterior superior iliac spine was higher than the left, the right posterior superior iliac spine was lower than the left, and the right anterior superior iliac spine was more lateral to the umbilicus than the left. Initial treatment included ice massage, stretch of the muscles in spasm, and mobilization of the sacroiliac and involved lumbar vertebral joints, which resolved the patient's pain and symptoms for up to 1 day, but then symptoms returned.

Discussion Questions

1. Why did the addition of the myofascial and positional-release therapy techniques assist with the effectiveness of the joint mobilization techniques?

2. Why would the resolution of shoulder instability impact the spasms in the trapezius and latissimus dorsi musculature?

3. If all of the spasms in the musculature were resolved following a treatment but the anomalies in the joints were not addressed by the therapy, what might you expect to occur once the patient became physically active again?

Resolution

After 4 weeks of treatment, with relief of symptoms lasting up to 2 days, it was decided to begin a more nontraditional treatment regimen, which included moist heat treatments over the paraspinal and latissimus dorsi muscles for 10 to 15 minutes, followed by myofascial release techniques for the paraspinal muscles, lower and middle trapezius, rhomboids, and latissimus dorsi muscle. A positional release technique was also used to treat the tender points on the same musculature, as well as those on the hip flexors, pectineus, lumbar and sacral spines, and piriformis. Mobilization of the sacroiliac joint and the involved lumbar spine joints was also performed. All treatments were followed by an application of an ice pack for 15 minutes. The patient's home program involved pelvic floor and thoracolumbar stability exercises, as well as a home program to improve the instability of the right shoulder and balance the strength and flexibility of the shoulder musculature. As shoulder strength improved and became more balanced, the positive effects of the sacroiliac joint and lumbosacral musculature treatments lasted longer, eventually decreasing the need for myofascial therapy and lessening the number of tender points to treat.

*Notes:*_____
_____
_____
_____
_____
_____

5

Domain V
Organizational and Professional Health and Well-Being

SCENARIO 1: EMERGENCY UTILIZATION OF SPORTS MEDICINE TEAM

At a college football game, an athlete received a traumatic elbow dislocation and was treated at the emergency department. After the athlete was released, the athlete reported pain at the wrist and, upon evaluation by the athletic trainer and confirmation through x-rays, it was further determined that the injured athlete had sustained a displaced scaphoid fracture, which required immediate care and possible surgery. The athletic trainer contacted the athlete's insurance company, which stated that the athlete would not have coverage for the office visit with the hand specialist because it was not an emergency admittance and was outside of the network area. The athlete had to return home to receive treatment and ensure full coverage benefits. The athlete was attending school 300 miles away from home and was not be able to travel to receive the treatment.

Discussion Questions

1. Who could the athletic trainer contact to help with the situation?

2. What steps could be taken to ensure proper care and insurance coverage?

3. Could anything have been done prior to the situation?

Gorse KM, Feld F, Blanc RO, eds.
Athletic Training Case Scenarios:
Domain-Based Situations and Solutions (pp 171-224).
© 2016 Taylor & Francis Group.

Resolution

The athletic trainer used the sports medicine team at the school by contacting the team physician who was affiliated with the hand specialist. The team physician explained the situation, and the hand specialist recommended having the athlete return to the emergency department and be admitted, where he would be on call for immediate care. Because the resultant visit was deemed an emergency admittance, the insurance company allowed the coverage for the care of the scaphoid injury.

*Notes:*_____

_____

_____

_____

_____

SCENARIO 2: MINOR CRISIS WITHIN A MAJOR SPORTING EVENT

An athletic trainer was part of the medical operations plan for a major sporting event as the Medical Operations Manager. During the event, an incident was reported via 911 of a possible bomb along the race course. The call was forwarded to the Director of Homeland Security within the city, who determined that it was not safe to continue the race along the designated course. The Director of Homeland Security communicated directly with the police officers along the race course to reroute the race prior to notifying race operations or the medical team. The athletic trainer (Medical Operations Manager) and the medical director were standing within the finish line area when several runners appeared to be advancing to the finish line against the direction of the intended race course. At the same time, they noticed that runners were also entering the finish line area in the intended finish line direction. It was later determined that there was no bomb and no threat to anyone's safety.

Discussion Questions

1. Do you think there is a threat to the runner's safety within the finish line with runners entering from 2 directions? Why or why not?

2. Who should be included in the crisis communications plan for the event?

3. Who is the final decision maker for security issues and potential threats during the event?

Resolution

The athletic trainer ran to the end of the street to see why the runners were advancing in the wrong direction. It appeared that a group of runners moved the street barricades and that everyone was following them. The athletic trainer communicated with the race operations team about what was happening, and staff was sent to the area to replace the barricades and reroute the runners back to the intended finish line area.

Additional Resolution

Since the event, a hierarchy of decision makers was put in place. Key personnel, including the Directors of Homeland Security, Police Chief, Race Director, Director of Logistics, and the Medical Director, were included in all decisions regarding the health and safety of runners and spectators. An emergency notification system was in place to alert runners, spectators, and volunteers via text message of any changes in the race course and all other necessary information. Snow fencing was in place along the finish line area so there was no confusion regarding which direction runners were to enter the finish line area.

Editor's Note

In the aftermath of the terrorist attacks of September 11, the need for a consistent incident command system was identified and the Federal Government established the National Incident Management System, which is currently used by all public safety agencies in the country. The National Incident Management System is a series of 6 courses that explain the system and stress the need for a unified command system so that all agencies working a large event are aware of actions taken by each other. Four of the courses can be completed online and all are free of charge. The 2 classroom courses are designed for supervisory personnel. Athletic trainers who are working events in conjunction with public safety agencies should take these classes to enhance their relationships and working experiences.

Notes:
_____
_____
_____
_____
_____
_____

SCENARIO 3: WORKING RELATIONSHIP BETWEEN ATHLETIC TRAINERS AND EMERGENCY MEDICAL SERVICES

An athletic trainer assessed a high school football player on the field who had sustained an axial load to the cervical spine during a varsity football game. The athlete reported moderate neck pain and some tingling going down both arms. All vital signs taken (pulse and respirations) were normal. There were signs of a possible cervical spine injury when the athletic trainer performed sensory and motor tests between C1 and T1. The athletic trainer determined that the local emergency medical services (EMS) stationed near the sidelines needed to be summoned onto the field to assist with the management of the injury. The EMS determined that the football helmet and shoulder pads must be removed for safe transport to the emergency care facility. The athletic trainer voiced his opinion based on training that it was safer to keep the helmet in place to avoid further injury. The consequence of the difference of opinions was that the EMS and the athletic trainer debated their points for several minutes while the athlete lay on the field.

Discussion Questions

1. Who has jurisdiction in this case? Why?

2. Do you think that the football helmet should be removed on the field before transport to the emergency facility? Why or why not?

3. What should have been done by the athletic trainer to prevent this situation from occurring?

Resolution

The athletic training staff and the EMS needed to work together in this situation and have a proper and legal emergency action plan (EAP) in place for the site/venue. This EAP was developed and practiced with all sports medicine team members, which included certified athletic trainers, student athletic trainers, team physicians, and local EMS.

*Notes:*_____

_____

_____

_____

_____

_____

SCENARIO 4: REDUCTION OF A TIBIOTALAR DISLOCATION BY NONMEDICAL PERSONNEL

While covering a wrestling tournament, I was called to a mat in which a 16-year-old male wrestling student athlete was lying face down and pounding his fists on the mat in obvious pain. As I approached the patient, I performed a quick survey of the scene and of the patient and noticed an obvious 180-degree dislocation of the right tibiotalar joint. Suddenly, as I approached the patient, the wrestling coach ran onto the mat, grabbed the patient's foot, and proceeded to twist it to relocate the dislocation. Before I could yell to stop the impending outcome, the coach had reduced the ankle. When I arrived at the patient, I asked the coach to step back as I began my primary evaluation. The patient had no tenderness to palpation over the shaft of the tibia or fibula, and palpation of the medial and lateral malleoli resulted in no abnormal tenderness. In addition, there was no obvious fracture or continued dislocation. I removed the patient's shoe and sock and noticed that he had immediate swelling around the tibiotalar joint, and the skin was warm to the touch. Proximal and distal pulses, neurological screen, and capillary refill were all within normal limits. Compression test of the tibia and fibula, Tinel's sign over the shafts of the tibia and fibula, and heel strike test were all negative for pain. The patient was then immobilized and referred to the emergency room for further evaluation.

Discussion Questions

1. How would you discuss/address your concerns in this situation with the coach, and in which setting would you choose to have the discussion (ie, office, hallway, gymnasium)?

2. Would you inform the athletic director or administration of the coach's actions? Why or why not? Because the student athlete is a minor, do you have a legal obligation to inform the parents of the coach's actions? Why or why not?

3. As an athletic trainer, what steps or actions could you implement to try and prevent an incident such as this from occurring?

Resolution

After the incident, I approached the wrestling coach and asked if he had any medical training. He stated he had not, other than a first aid and cardiopulmonary resuscitation course through the Red Cross. When asked why he would perform such an action as to reduce a serious injury such as a dislocation, he responded with, "Because I couldn't stand looking at the injury." I informed him that it would be beneficial for the health and safety of all participants if he would use the skills he has only been properly trained to perform.

Additional Resolution

In reflecting upon this situation, there are several steps I could have performed prior to the incident to perhaps prevent an incident like this one from occurring. Prior to the tournament, there was no extensive meeting held with the coaches, medical staff, and tournament officials regarding EAPs and procedures other than to review skin check policies and the location of medical staff and equipment. An EAP is only effective if all parties are privy to the information, it is reviewed, and all parties have a clear and concise knowledge of their responsibilities during an incident. Secondly, the wrestling event was severely understaffed. There was one athletic trainer and 3 athletic training students, as well as 2 emergency medical technicians (EMTs) for 12 mats of competition. Although response time to each mat was less than 20 seconds, having more staff at the event could have allowed medical personnel to intervene prior to the coach reaching the student athlete.

Notes:_____

_____

_____

_____

_____

_____

SCENARIO 5: SUSPECTED DRUG USE IN AN ATHLETE

The athletic trainer at a small college was assigned to care for several sports teams, one of which was the crew team, which was co-ed. One day, one of the male rowers asked to meet with the athletic trainer about a concern he had about one of his teammates, a 20-year-old female. He explained that he and the female had been friends for a few years and often hung out with the same group of friends on the weekends. He explained that she used to use drugs, specifically cocaine, but that she had been clean for more than 1 year. However, the other day, he had stopped by her dorm room to ask for some notes from a class they were in together and noticed that she was acting very odd, just like she acted when she was on cocaine previously. He asked her if she was using again, but she just told him to go away and leave her alone. The male rower was very concerned about her.

Two days later, another teammate went to see the athletic trainer to state that she had also noticed very erratic behavior in the female rower on a few occasions over the past couple of weeks and also thought that she was using cocaine again. The athletic trainer spoke to the coach and asked if he had noticed any unusual behavior in any of his athletes in the past 1 or 2 months that would make him suspect that any of them were using illegal drugs. The coach told him that he had not seen anything unusual and that the team was doing quite well lately.

Discussion Questions

1. How will you decide whether you have enough information to warrant a drug test based on reasonable suspicion?

2. With whom should you discuss/not discuss this issue? What principles will guide this decision?

3. Should you meet with the female rower to get her side of the story before requiring her to submit to a drug test? Why or why not?

Resolution

The athletic trainer discussed the issue with another staff athletic trainer, who felt that this was not enough evidence to require a drug test. However, the athletic trainer had seen a close family member struggle with drug addiction and felt he had to try to help the athlete who might be in trouble. The athletic trainer decided not to confront the female rower because he was sure that she would just deny the drug use and have too much time to prepare for a drug test. In addition, the athletic trainer learned that the university did not have a policy regarding drug testing of athletes based on reasonable suspicion. The athletic trainer called the athlete's parents to express his concerns. Her parents took her for a drug test, which was negative, and reported the athletic trainer's inappropriate actions to the university administration. The administration reprimanded the athletic trainer for contacting her parents because she was no longer a minor. The athletic trainer also learned that the athlete who had initially reported her unusual behavior was her ex-boyfriend, who had been stalking her.

Additional Resolution

If the athletic trainer could do it over again, he would do several things differently:

1. Meet with the head athletic trainer and athletic director for advice and follow it.

2. Meet with the female athlete to allow her to give her side of the story.

3. Not call her parents, as this was a violation of the athlete's privacy.

4. Recognize his overreaction to the situation because of his personal family history.

5. Thoroughly document each meeting immediately following the meeting.

Notes:_____

_____

_____

_____

_____

SCENARIO 6: RELEASE OF LIABILITY AGAINST A DOCTOR'S RECOMMENDATION

An athletic trainer had assessed a high school women's lacrosse player who had presented with signs and symptoms synonymous with a stress reaction or stress fracture. The athlete was referred to an orthopedic surgeon for further testing and treatment where she had a series of x-rays to rule out a bone fracture. All x-rays were negative. The athlete was scheduled for a magnetic resonance imaging (MRI) test.

Upon completion of the physician visit, the athlete was instructed to restrict all sports participation until the completion and results of the MRI came in. After the physician visit, the parents and athlete were unhappy with the recommendations of the orthopedic surgeon. The athlete wanted to compete in an interscholastic athletic competition before the completion of the MRI. The athletic trainer would not allow participation because of the orthopedic surgeon's recommendation and pending diagnosis.

The parents presented the athletic trainer with a written note that released the athletic trainer, orthopedic surgeon, and school district of any liability if the athlete participated against physician recommendation.

Discussion Questions

1. Is the parental release from liability permissible for the athlete's participation? Why?

2. Do you think there are any legal ramifications with which the athletic trainer should have been concerned? Why or why not?

3. Should the school superintendent and solicitor be consulted for this type of situation?

Resolution

Upon completion of conversation with a school administrator, the athlete was allowed to participate in the interscholastic event. The note was copied and distributed to the head athletic trainer, orthopedic physician, school athletic director, and the athlete's athletic file.

*Notes:*_____

_____

_____

_____

_____

SCENARIO 7: HANDLING CHALLENGES FROM COACHING STAFF PERSONNEL

A newly certified athletic trainer was the home athletic trainer at a rescheduled college softball game that was being played on a Sunday afternoon. There were no other events going on and no additional sports medicine staff. An opposing player hit a possible triple and was running around second base. The athlete went down and was screaming and holding her right knee. The home athletic trainer ran out to assess the athlete and concluded that the athlete had no end feel with ligamentous testing of the right lateral knee. The away coach came out and told the athletic trainer that this athlete had no pain tolerance and that she was fine. They did not have any sports medicine staff with them, although the head coach did allow the assistant coach to help the athletic trainer remove the athlete from the field. The injured softball player's knee was treated with ice, elevation, a compression wrap, and an immobilizer. The athlete was from a college 2 hours away, which was also close to her home. She was medically stable and asked the athletic trainer to allow her to go to her home emergency room/physician. Crutch instruction was given, but the athlete had too much discomfort to ambulate a functional distance. The softball field was 350 yards from the athletic training room/field house, and the athletic trainer only had a large push cart for supplies. At the end of the game, the away coaching staff insisted that the injured athlete did not need assistance and they did not appreciate the severity of the athlete's injury despite extensive education by the home athletic trainer. The home athletic trainer removed all supplies from the cart and was able to safely move the athlete back up to the field house with the help of a home junior varsity player. The home athletic trainer was able to get the injured player into their college van without assistance from her coaches and elevated the right leg with fresh ice. The player and the coaches were given final instructions, and the athlete's mother was called by the home athletic trainer about the athlete's injury, estimated arrival time, and recommendations.

Discussion Questions

1. Should the athletic trainer have just called EMS for proper transport from the field? Why or why not?

2. Does the away player's coach supersede the decision of the home athletic trainer who does not have an established relationship with the athlete?

3. Was there a better choice to help the athletic trainer transport the player from the field to the field house other than the junior varsity player?

Resolution

This athletic trainer did an appropriate evaluation of this athlete and provided proper first aid care and treatment despite being a new graduate. It is unfortunate to be challenged by someone who has an established relationship with the athlete and should also respect the knowledge of an athletic trainer. The athletic trainer still has the responsibility for providing proper medical care for all athletes, home and away, if they are the only providers present. Athletic trainers need to have confidence in their decisions and provide the care that is appropriate for athletes regardless of what coaches say or want athletic trainers to do.

Additional Resolution

Three days later, an assistant coach from the away team came to the home athletic trainer's field house to return the immobilizer and crutches. She also had a thank you card from the head coach because this athlete required surgery to repair the lateral complex of her right knee.

Notes:_____
_____
_____
_____
_____
_____

SCENARIO 8: PROTECTING ATHLETES' INFORMATION ON SOCIAL MEDIA

A Division III college had a blog site where students could discuss all aspects of college activities. A student blogged about how bad the football team was lately and how he was embarrassed to go to their games. There was significant activity on the blog site, and another student posted that the team was not in good enough shape and had to train harder. A student, who was in the athletic training program, posted that the team was doing poorly because of injuries, not because they had not trained. He stated that in 2 weeks, the team should be better because the tight end was recovering well from his left knee medial collateral ligament tear and the wide receiver did not have a fracture and would be able to play with his fingers taped together. The athletic trainer student posted that one of the offensive lineman was still definitely out because he had a lumbar herniated disk.

A senior athletic training student saw the blog and immediately called the sophomore student and told him to stop blogging this information. The sophomore athletic training student told the senior student that there was no problem because he had not blogged the athletes' full names. The senior athletic training student contacted his supervising athletic trainer to let her know that the information was present on social media. The athletic trainer stopped the blog activity, and an investigation began regarding the sophomore student exposing athlete's private information on social media.

Discussion Questions

1. Was the consequence too severe for this infraction since this was his first offense?

2. Why was there a problem if no full names were given?

3. Does your school have a policy regarding social media and taking pictures during practice and games? Why or why not?

Resolution

The sophomore athletic training student was removed from the Athletic Training Program on the grounds that, before students are allowed to observe or participate in an athlete's care, they are given extensive education on privacy and protected information and must sign a confidentiality agreement.

The student was removed from their Athletic Training Program because he had been familiarized with the requirements for individuals working in health care. All individuals, whether they are office staff, students, or athletic trainers, have the responsibility to maintain confidentiality about their athlete's information and medical status. The sophomore student felt that he was defending the team, but there was too much to identify the athletes, even without their full names given. Personnel in the athletic training setting have access to privileged information that has to be protected at all times.

*Notes:*_____

_____

_____

_____

_____

_____

SCENARIO 9: JUSTIFYING ATHLETIC TRAINING WITHIN TOUGH FINANCIAL TIMES

The Dean of the School of Health and Human Performance, which houses the Athletic Training Program, attended a Kinesiology Department faculty meeting to address the topic of significant financial difficulties within the college. Due to recent decreases in state funding, the college had become significantly more dependent on tuition revenue than in previous years. This necessitated a change in the enrollment model that the college had traditionally used. This traditional model relied heavily on state support, with very little dependency on enrollment and tuition revenue. As a result of the new reliance on tuition funds, the proposed model would potentially eliminate programs with low enrollment and invest in programs that demonstrated high levels of quality, those with large enrollments, or programs with the potential to increase enrollment based on workforce demands. Programs that could demonstrate the potential to grow and attract quality students would receive significant new resources (new faculty lines, equipment, etc) from the college. To begin to address this issue, the administration would examine the enrollment, success, staffing, and current faculty workloads for all majors within the school. Future staffing and workload would be dependent on the current and projected enrollment of each major. Majors demonstrating low enrollment or overstaffing were to be subjected to faculty reductions and/or elimination of the major.

The Athletic Training Program was identified as a major with low enrollment by the administration despite its accredited status and high-quality students. The director of the Athletic Training Program was tasked with justifying the current status of the major and demonstrating the potential to expand enrollment within athletic training.

Discussion Questions

1. What steps would you take to justify the low enrollment in the Athletic Training Program?

2. What types of data could you collect to demonstrate the quality and success of the Athletic Training Program?

3. How would you go about campaigning for an increase in faculty for the Athletic Training Program?

Resolution

The first step in the resolution of this situation was the collection of data to justify the existence of the Athletic Training Program. A major point in justification was demonstrating that the perceived low enrollment in the major was due to accreditation standards. The president of the college was a huge proponent of national accreditations, and we made it a point to promote our Commission on Accreditation of Athletic Training Education accreditation and the standards that were mandated by accreditation. When including the Athletic Training Intent major with the Athletic Training Program, the total number of students was significantly higher than at first glance. The second piece of data that we collected was information regarding the high school grade point averages, standardized test scores, and college grade point averages of athletic training majors. These data demonstrated that the athletic training majors at the college were among the highest achieving students admitted and attending the college. We also provided data demonstrating the success of athletic training majors on the Board of Certification, including examination and in admission to graduate schools across the country. Finally, we provided data demonstrating the workload of the athletic training faculty. These data demonstrated that the faculty within the major accounted for an extremely high number of full-time equivalents. The number of full-time equivalents/faculty members generated exceeded any other major on campus.

After review of all of the data provided, the administration decided that the Athletic Training Program was a valuable asset to the college and that there was a great deal of potential to expand and provide additional resources to support the major.

Notes:_____

_____

_____

_____

_____

_____

SCENARIO 10: TIME TO TAKE A STAND

One Friday night during a varsity football game with our biggest rival, late in the third quarter, our defensive back got in position to make a tackle and, at the last second, ducked his head. I have seen this hundreds of times before as an athletic trainer. Each time I see this, I talk to the athlete about the importance of keeping his head up. I was already formulating what I was going to say to this athlete when I noticed he was not getting up or moving. Both were immediate signals that we had a potentially serious injury on our hands. As the team physician and I ran onto the field, I examined the surroundings and the athlete; there were no issues with the field, there were no gross deformities, and the athlete was breathing but not conscious. I immediately moved to the head and stabilized the head/helmet between my forearms.

Our team physician started trying to awaken the athlete. Fortunately, the player came to rather quickly, and we were able to check his vital signs and start asking questions. He had pain in his neck near the center of the spine, tingling and numbness in all 4 extremities, and a burning sensation running down his spine at the time of contact. The physician called the EMS onto the field. While they were bringing their equipment onto the field, the physician and I worked together on stabilizing the head and neck and completing a sensory distribution test. Through sensory and motor tests, it was decided that this athlete had a cervical spine injury near C2 through C5. We relayed this information to the rescue personnel, and they immediately wanted to remove the helmet. His breathing was not compromised or labored and he was awake and responsive, so there was no need at that time to remove the helmet. I also knew through my years of schooling and working with football that there was no way the helmet should be removed. I started to discuss proper protocol with regard to football equipment, and they wanted to hear none of it. They stated that they had a protocol that they had to follow and since we summoned them onto the field that they were now in charge of the situation. It was not the time or place to discuss protocol or equipment issues, so I asked my team physician to please take a stand. He said, "Do not remove the helmet!" Their response was, "That is fine, but you need to accompany the athlete to the hospital," to which he immediately stated, "Fine, let's pack him up and get going." At that time, we did a lift onto the spine board with my athletic training student aides and other EMS assisting. Because I was at the head and stabilizing the athlete's cervical spine, I was in charge, and the process went smoothly. The athlete was very cooperative and did not try to fight the process, something that is critical in those situations. Once secured on the spine board and on the gurney, transport to the local emergency department was uneventful. By the time they arrived at the hospital, the athlete had started to regain some sensation in his fingers and toes.

At the hospital, the equipment was removed methodically and correctly, which helped with the success of the situation. After the computed tomography scan, it was determined that the athlete had no fracture, no dislocation, and no concussion. Formal diagnosis was a spinal cord contusion, which explained the temporary paresthesia. The athlete made a full recovery within 2 days and returned to football within 2 weeks with no issues.

Discussion Questions

1. Should the equipment have stayed on during the transportation to the emergency department? Why or why not?

2. Do you feel that this situation was handled correctly? Why or why not? What could have been done to avoid this situation?

3. Describe the National Athletic Trainers Association's (NATA's) position statement on equipment removal in football.

Resolution

The day after this situation was presented, I began discussions with the director of the local rescue service. This effort resulted in a yearly in-service with all employees. This educational seminar used the staff licensed athletic trainers to train in the equipment used in all of our sports. We practiced the spine boarding techniques and our protocols. This has expanded to protocols with exertional heat illness and our EAPs for all venues, and resulted in a cooperative environment between the 2 emergency health care professionals. We have also shared equipment with them in regard to football helmet facemask removal that they could use while providing emergency care to the local midget football league.

Notes:_____

_____

_____

_____

_____

_____

SCENARIO 11: TO TREAT OR NOT TO TREAT

You were an athletic trainer traveling with an intercollegiate baseball team for an out-of-state game. The state you were traveling to required licensing to practice as an athletic trainer, which you did not have. The host athletic trainer was covering another game off campus 10 minutes away but was in contact via walkie talkie. Between innings, a student spectator sitting behind first base was hit in the face by an overthrown baseball. You were called over by the first base umpire. Upon arriving, you noticed a large vertical laceration extending from the nasal bone to the maxilla. There was a perfuse epistaxis with nasal deformity. The student was conscious but exhibiting signs of shock.

Discussion Questions

1. As an athletic trainer not licensed to practice in the state you are visiting, are you required to treat this individual? Why or why not?

2. Who is responsible for initiating EMS—the umpire, the visiting athletic trainer, or the host athletic trainer?

3. What is a Good Samaritan Law and does it apply to this circumstance? What care can be provided under this law? Does this law vary by state?

Resolution

It is the responsibility of the visiting athletic trainer to familiarize his- or herself with a particular state's regulations specific to the practice of athletic training. Certain states grant licensing to treat athletes only. Other states may have an exemption in its licensing act that allows a visiting athletic trainer to work with his or her own team in providing care (J. Barker, personal communication; J. Pulice, personal communication, April 8, 2014, respectively).

*Notes:*_____

_____

_____

_____

_____

_____

SCENARIO 12: SOCCER HEADING THE BALL COLLISION

An athletic trainer and a student first responder, who was a registered EMT, were covering a home soccer game. There was a collision on the field when 2 players went up to head the ball. One athlete was on the ground lying supine, grabbing his head and yelling in pain. The other athlete had a minor bleeding laceration above his right eyebrow.

The athletic trainer began to interview the athlete on the ground and established manual in-line stabilization while the student EMT attended to the bleeding facial laceration. The athletic trainer activated the facility EAP, and EMS was summoned. The other player was stabilized and escorted to the sidelines by the coach. The student EMT came over and took over manual stabilization so the athletic trainer could further assess the athlete on the ground. As the athletic trainer was checking motor and sensory function of the lower extremities, a visiting team's parent from the bleachers walked up, said he was a doctor, and insisted the athlete was okay. The game official agreed, and he and the doctor pulled the athlete into a sitting position, and the doctor and the visiting team coach walked the athlete to the visitor's bench. The athlete sat on the bench holding his head.

The EMS unit arrived and was escorted to the visitor's bench by the facility manager, who met them at the entrance to the field. A loud argument ensued between the doctor and EMS personnel. The EMS came over and started yelling at the athletic trainer and the student EMT and asked, "Why was the athlete moved?"

Discussion Questions

1. Who has jurisdiction in this case, the athletic trainer or EMS? Why? What could the athletic trainer have done/said to prevent this situation from occurring?

2. What policies could be put into place to help better navigate a situation like this in the future?

3. Should officials and coaches be briefed before competition on the chain of command for an injury occurrence? If so, what would be the best means for this type of communication?

Resolution

After the game, the student EMT and athletic trainer sat down and discussed what occurred and what could have been done differently.

The athletic trainer met with the head team physician and athletic director to discuss concerns regarding someone coming out of the stands and taking control of the situation. The team physician insisted that the policy be that the athletic trainer has say regarding the care of the injured athlete regardless of who is in attendance, only deferring to the team physician if he or she is in attendance.

There was a discussion with the soccer coaches, as well as the game officials, prior to the next home game to clarify the protocol and procedure for caring for an injury on the field.

Notes:_____

_____

_____

_____

_____

_____

SCENARIO 13: OUTREACH
HIGH SCHOOL ATHLETIC TRAINER

An athletic trainer was working as an outreach athletic trainer at a local high school for the year. During the summer months, the high school baseball team had games during the late afternoon. The athletic trainer was required to be there early in the morning and through the afternoon for all other summer camps that were in session during the summer. After talking to the head baseball coach, the athletic trainer was told that athletic trainers did not need to be there for the games as long as they provided water. The head coach said if there was an injury, most likely they would have to activate the EAP and call for EMS. The athletic trainer asked for a game schedule from the head coach.

A few weeks after the discussion with the head coach, there was an injury during a game. A visiting team athlete was struck in the nose with a baseball. The result was an epistaxis. The athletic director of the high school called over the radio for the athletic trainer on coverage that day. There was no response. The athletic director brought the athlete down to the athletic training room, and there was no one there.

The next day, the athletic director summoned the athletic trainer into her office. The athletic director asked why there was no coverage at the previous day's baseball game. The athletic trainer explained that the head baseball coach said that all the games did not need to be covered earlier in the summer and that all they wanted was water for the games. The athletic trainer also said that they asked the coach for a game schedule multiple times and no schedule was produced. The athletic director told the athletic trainer that all games must be covered for the remainder of the summer. The athletic trainer never received a schedule for the remaining games of the summer.

Discussion Questions

1. What other questions should have been brought up by the athletic trainer to the head coach when he said no athletic trainer was needed during games?

2. What other actions should the athletic trainer have taken to make sure that not being present at any baseball games was okay?

3. What information regarding roles and responsibilities should be included in an outreach contract?

Resolution

The athletic director asked the athletic trainer's employer at the local clinic to remove the athletic trainer from the high school after this incident. There were other incidents that were involved in this decision; the athletic trainer supported this decision because the athletic director asked for too much outside of athletic training job responsibilities. No other facts are known about this scenario because the athletic trainer left the high school.

*Notes:*_____

_____

_____

_____

_____

_____

SCENARIO 14: IS A POLICY AND PROCEDURE MANUAL HELPFUL?

A newly certified athletic trainer interviewed with the athletic administrator and assistant principal of a high school that had not employed an athletic trainer in the recent past. He accepted the offer for a position as that school's athletic trainer and reported 2 days prior to the first day of summer practice for fall sports. The athletic trainer met with the head coaches for the fall sports and introduced himself, provided a quick overview of his background, and reviewed his thoughts on what he would cover and when and what services he would provide, etc.

He approached his new job using his policy and procedures manual he developed as his administration class assignment. Things went well for a few weeks as he took notes on what small issues arose that he felt he should have a more substantial directive in writing and planned to complete it when things settled down.

Then, the star running back got his hand smashed between 2 helmets during a practice the day before a big game with a district rival. The athlete presented with swelling and point tenderness over the third and fourth metacarpals with crepitus. The athletic trainer said, to the parent, "You must see a physician before he can play; I believe there is a good chance his hand is fractured."

The parent agreed to take the athlete to a physician after the game and told him to tape it up for the game.

The athlete returned to school on game day with a note from the physician that said "approved to participate with tape for game on (date indicated)." After discussing the physician visit with the athlete, he acknowledged that he did not get an x-ray and that the physician who provided the note was a friend of his father. When this was brought up to the athletic administrator, he argued that a note was required from a physician and that the athlete had a note, so the athletic trainer should let him play.

Discussion Questions

1. Create a list of all the policies and procedures that you should have written and approved by your employer prior to beginning an athletic training job.

2. Explain your response to a request of a signed statement from the parents of the athlete in this type of situation identifying the risks involved in participation in football with an unstable metacarpal fracture. Would you consider this a reasonable response?

3. Is there any tape job that you would consider acceptable to use that would allow this high school athlete to safely continue to play in a varsity game?

Resolution

This situation is common among young athletic trainers entering the workforce for the first time. Having a policy and procedures manual that addresses the essentials provides support for the athletic trainer to be able to provide the appropriate care and ensure the safety of every athlete participating in sports under their watch. What is often forgotten is that this manual should be developed with input from the coaches, school administration, and the physician who provides direction to the athletic trainer. It is also essential that the policies and procedures go through an approval process within the school's hierarchy, so when the less-than-popular decision must be made, the emotions of a particular event will not cloud doing the right thing to protect the safety and well-being of the athlete.

Additional Resolution

Developing policies and procedures prior to needing them is essential for athletic trainers to maintain a sense of security and support in their decisions when the unfortunate happens. This concept should begin with the job interview; a question that the candidate should ask the potential employers is, "What are your policies and procedures for...?" and then fill in the blanks, from return-to-play to heat protocols, weight loss in wrestling, coverage policy, travel policy, team physician, hydration protocol, infectious disease prevention, automated external defibrillator policy, etc.

Notes:_____

_____

_____

_____

_____

SCENARIO 15: RELEASE OF PROTECTED HEALTH INFORMATION FOR CONSULTING REPORT

A sports medicine manager was instructed to meet with a consulting group to assess the sports medicine division of the orthopedic service-line within the health care organization. One of the consultants asked the manager to send protected health information to them through the consulting company's e-mail address. After discussing the request with another department administrator, you found that the consulting group did not have an executed Business Associates Agreement (BAA) in place.

When approached to submit a BAA, the consultant said that the information was required immediately to generate the findings report. The consultant noted a short-term consulting agreement, in lieu of a BAA, was already agreed upon between the entities and that any delays in the relay of information could make the health system liable for additional fees. The sports medicine manager apologized for the delay, declined the consultant's request, and delayed the process reporting.

Discussion Questions

1. Should the manager have transferred the data to save the health system money?

2. When there is a question in policy, who should decide procedure?

3. What is a BAA and why is it important to have an executed agreement?

Resolution

The administrator contacted the Chief Information Officer of the health system and requested approval to transfer information. The Chief Information Officer explained that the consulting company had not yet executed the BAA. In addition, the consulting group needed to have a temporary e-mail account set up to protect all information sent through electronic files. No information could be e-mailed until proper procedure was in place by the health system and consulting group.

*Notes:*_____

_____

_____

_____

_____

_____

SCENARIO 16: STUDENT ATHLETE INJURY REFERRAL

Upon your evaluation of a student athlete's knee, you determined that a referral to the orthopedic surgeon was necessary. At this college, a physician was not readily available in the athletic training clinic, so the athletic trainer had to make an appointment for the student athlete. Once the call was made and the receptionist viewed the scheduling computer, you were asked about the patient.

Discussion Questions

1. To establish the appointment in a timely manner, what patient documents would you need in front of you?

2. Do you need written permission from the athlete to make an appointment?

3. Is there a better way to handle student athlete referrals to physicians for medical evaluations? If so, what is a better way to handle situations like this one?

Resolution

The following must be included in a student athlete medical file/chart:
- Class schedule: try not to set an appointment during classes
- Personal data: date of birth, permanent address, phone number, etc
- Student's personal medical insurance card and photo identification
- University excess/secondary athletic accident insurance

*Notes:*_____

_____

_____

_____

_____

_____

SCENARIO 17: ATHLETIC TRAINING PROGRAM CLOSURE

A program director of an accredited program received a call from her dean on her cell phone at 7 o'clock at night. The dean was calling to inform the doctor that the university had instituted significant budget cuts for the next academic year. As a result, the dean was going to propose closure of the Athletic Training Program to balance the budget. The dean explained that her proposal would have to be approved by the provost, the faculty senate, and then the board of trustees. The dean instructed the doctor to work with the Associate Dean of Administrative Affairs to put together a counterproposal. It was university policy that any program being considered for closure had the opportunity to submit a counterproposal. The counterproposal should include documented evidence for the need of the program, documented evidence that the program is critical to the mission of the university, and documented evidence of financial viability of the program.

The doctor got to work immediately because she was going on maternity leave in 3 weeks. She scheduled a joint meeting with the Associate Dean of Administrative Affairs and the Director of Budget for her unit to start compiling the necessary documents for the counterproposal. Meanwhile, she launched a letter writing campaign in support of the Athletic Training Program. She had students, alumni, athletic trainers, coaches, and other community partners write personal letters to the dean, provost, and president of the university. This infuriated the dean. The dean called her into his office to express his displeasure with her actions. He had expected her to work quietly on the counterproposal.

The doctor completed the counterproposal prior to going on maternity leave. During the development of the counterproposal, she was able to establish a valuable alliance with the Associate Dean of Administrative Affairs and the Director of Budget. Together, they monitored the situation and kept the doctor in the know. The proposal for closure of the program was approved by the provost. While on maternity leave, the doctor presented the counterproposal to the faculty senate. As a result, the faculty senate did not support the closure of the program. The board of trustees also did not support the closure of the program. The counterproposal worked!

One month later, the athletic training program was about to admit students to the next incoming class. To the doctor's surprise, she received an e-mail from the provost instructing her not to admit students. She quickly replied to the provost asking why she was not to admit students. He informed her that recent data sent to him from the dean indicated that the program was operating $50,000 in the red. The doctor cut her maternity leave short and returned to work. In collaboration with the Associate Dean of Administrative Affairs and the Director of Budget, she conducted a thorough review of the budget and submitted evidence to the provost that the program was not operating in the red. The provost directed the dean and the doctor to work together to resolve the inconsistencies in the budget data.

Discussion Questions

1. What information would you include in the counterproposal to justify the need for the athletic training program?

2. How would you have demonstrated the financial viability of the athletic training program?

3. Would you have handled the situation differently? If so, how?

Resolution

In a joint meeting with the dean, the Associate Dean of Administrative Affairs, the Director of Budget, and the doctor, the budget inconsistencies were resolved. The program was not operating in the red. The correct budget information was provided to the provost, and the doctor was permitted to admit a new class.

Since the proposed closure of the program, a new dean was hired, who fully supports the athletic training program.

*Notes:*_____

_____

_____

_____

_____

_____

Scenario 18: Accreditation Violation

A program director of an accredited Athletic Training Program received a phone call from an alumna of his program at 4:10 on a Friday evening. The alumna called to inform the program director that a current student from his program just arrived to her athletic training facility to cover the 7:00 night baseball game scheduled between their institutions. The alumna was concerned because the student traveled with the baseball team without an athletic trainer/preceptor, and she knew this was a violation of the program's direct supervision policy. She offered to supervise the student during the baseball game, although she was not a trained preceptor. The program director thanked her for letting him know and ended the telephone call to address the issue.

The program director immediately called the student's assigned preceptor. The program director was concerned because he was aware that the baseball team left on Wednesday for a 3-game road trip. When he got in touch with the preceptor, she informed him that there was a last-minute change in her schedule that prevented her from traveling with the baseball team. She had decided to let the student go on the trip because she thought it would be a great learning opportunity for him to travel with the baseball team. Also, the baseball coach really wanted the student to travel with the team as a reward for his hard work.

Discussion Questions

1. If you were the program director, what would your immediate course of action be in this case?

2. If you were the student in this case, how would you have handled this situation?

3. The direct supervision policy was violated in this case. What should the consequence(s) be for the student? The preceptor?

Resolution

The program director called the student directly to address the situation. He instructed the student that he was not permitted to touch (treat, stretch, etc) an athlete, he was not to sit in the dugout, and that he was to return home immediately. The program director documented the conversation via an e-mail summary of the verbal conversation. He also required the preceptor to communicate the same to the baseball coach, which was also documented via an e-mail summary of the verbal conversation. The baseball coach also replied via e-mail and noted his understanding of the situation. He also expressed his concern for the student in that he hoped this incident would not negatively affect his position in the Athletic Training Program.

The program director consulted with his Clinical Education Coordinator to develop a course of action. They held a formal meeting with the student and the preceptor. The preceptor was suspended for the remainder of the semester. She was required to attend additional clinical preceptor training prior to receiving another athletic training student. The student was also suspended from the clinical setting for 2 weeks, had to write a 20-page paper on ethical decision-making practices in athletic training, and had to provide an oral presentation of the incident to all students in the athletic training program. This presentation detailed his thoughts and decisions leading up to the incident, as well as the consequences he faced as a result of the situation.

Additional Resolution

We have a formal policy in place for students who practice "Unsafe or Unprofessional Athletic Training Practice" that outlines possible consequences if they violate this policy. However, we do not have a formal policy for preceptors related to this policy. Having a formal policy for preceptors would have facilitated our course of action in regard to the preceptor in question. We are in the process of creating a formal policy and procedure manual specifically for preceptors to address issues such as the one presented in this case.

Notes:_____

_____

_____

_____

_____

SCENARIO 19: UNPROFESSIONAL BEHAVIOR ACCUSATION

A female athletic trainer, who graduated from a professional Master of Science in Athletic Training Degree Program, accepted a head athletic trainer position at a large Texas high school upon graduation. She was eager to build a caring, professional reputation among the administrators, coaches, parents, and student athletes. She regularly baked cupcakes that she made available (at no charge) in the athletic training facility and during booster meetings. Although she was required to travel with the football team, she regularly traveled with other teams as well. She also wanted to get involved with teaching and mentoring students interested in athletic training, so she started an athletic training club. The athletic training club primarily consisted of female high school students who wanted to work with the successful football program. She began to have issues with one female high school student. It was evident that the student did not have an interest in athletic training; however, she was interested in interacting with the football players. The athletic trainer felt as though she could not address this situation with the student because her dad was the assistant athletic director.

At the end of the football season, the athletic trainer was called into the athletic director's office. He informed her that there were several complaints from members of the athletic training club regarding her unprofessional behavior, which was making the football players uncomfortable. He indicated that he interviewed several football players who felt as though she touched them inappropriately during clinical evaluations. The athletic director informed her that he had statements from 3 football players indicating that the felt uncomfortable when she evaluated their injuries. The athletic director gave her 2 options: (1) resign effective immediately or (2) be subject to an investigation that would likely result in her termination.

Discussion Questions

1. The athletic trainer has 2 options. Which would you chose and why?

2. What could the athletic trainer have done to avoid this situation?

3. How may the athletic trainer prove her innocence?

Resolution

The athletic trainer decided to resign because she felt as though she would not be able to provide evidence to support her professional behavior. She felt as though it was a "he said, she said" situation. She suspected that the female student was behind the accusations and that she convinced the football players to corroborate her story. The athletic trainer felt as though the situation would not be resolved in her favor, especially since the female student's dad was the assistant athletic director.

Additional Resolution

The athletic trainer probably should have taken time to get to know the administrators, coaches, parents, student athletes, and students, as well as to learn the political environment of the high school. More importantly, she should have developed policies and procedures for her athletic training facility, her professional practice, and the athletic training club.

Notes:_____

_____

_____

_____

_____

_____

SCENARIO 20: MEDICAL AUTHORITY FOR RETURN TO PLAY

A female collegiate swimmer suffered an asthmatic episode of moderate severity during her training session the day before an important competition. She was evaluated and treated by the primary care team physician, who prescribed anti-asthmatic medications. She was instructed to refrain from exercise for at least 3 days until her airway reactivity resolved. She was also instructed to have her lung function measured with a handheld spirometer by the athletic trainer every day until her follow-up with the physician the following week. The athletic trainer informed the coach of the physician's prescription and the athlete's activity restrictions. The coach listened carefully and had no questions for the athletic trainer. The athlete came back the following day to have her lung function assessed. Peak expiratory flow rate was 20% below predicted. The athlete was reminded to use her medications as prescribed and to avoid exercise.

The next morning, the athletic trainer read in the newspaper that the athlete had participated in the swimming competition. He called the athlete to ask how she was feeling and to find out why she competed against physician's orders. She replied that the coach gave her an over-the-counter inhaler to use, told her that she would be fine, and entered her in the swim meet. The athletic trainer was upset that the coach defied the college's duly appointed team physician and put the athlete's well-being at risk despite a clear and open channel of communication and an established protocol. When confronted later that day by the athletic trainer, the coach asserted that because he had asthma, he felt he knew how it should be handled with the athlete. Furthermore, the competition was an important one, and he did not want the athlete to be disappointed by being withheld from participation. When the athletic trainer reminded the coach that there was an established medical chain of authority for making return-to-play decisions, the coach indicated that he had no intention of being bound by such a policy. Upset, the athletic trainer informed the athletic director, and she intervened with the coach and insisted that he adhere to the medical chain of authority in the future. The athletic trainer informed her that if she failed to intervene in the matter, he would inform her supervisor.

Discussion Questions

1. What options could the athletic trainer in this situation have considered in addition to or as substitutes for the actions he took? What are the risks and rewards of approaching the athletic director with this matter?

2. Should the team physician be brought into this conflict with the coach? Why or why not?

3. Are you aware of instances of athletic trainer–coach conflict regarding medical management of an athlete's health and well-being? In what ways are your examples similar to the one described here? How are they different? Are there principles that apply across all conflicts of this type?

Resolution

The following day, the athletic director informed the athletic trainer that she had spoken with the coach and informed him of his responsibility to work within the medical chain of authority. She asserted that the situation should be resolved, but the athletic trainer and the coach never again established a basis of trust in dealing with injured or ill athletes. It is unclear if the coach's annual performance evaluation made any reference to the incident. The athlete recovered without further incident and successfully managed her asthma using the protocol prescribed by the physician.

Notes:_____

_____

_____

_____

_____

_____

SCENARIO 21: PROMOTING DIVERSITY IN ATHLETIC TRAINING

You recently attended a session at the NATA Annual Meeting sponsored by the Ethnic Diversity Advisory Committee that addressed the benefits of racial and ethnic diversity among the health care professions. You learned that, among these benefits, racial and ethnic minority health care providers are more likely to serve minority and medically underserved communities, thereby increasing access to care; racial and ethnic minority patients report greater levels of satisfaction with care provided by minority health care professionals; and racial and ethnic minority health care providers can help to reduce cultural and linguistic barriers and improve cultural competence. In short, the ethnic minority athletes and patients we treat benefit from being treated by people that look like themselves. At the lecture, you also learned that a dearth of ethnic minority athletic trainers exists to provide health care coverage to athletes and physically active patients in high schools, sports medicine clinics, colleges and universities, and professional sports. The presenter explained that more than 80% of the NATA membership is White, 2.6% is Black, 3% is Hispanic, and 3.6% is Asian or Pacific Islander. He also noted that approximately 35% of all athletes across all National Collegiate Athletic Association divisions are of color, and half of division I football and men's and women's basketball players are Black. You would like to contribute to diversifying the athletic training health care workforce but are unsure how you can help.

Discussion Questions

1. Say something about your life experience around this issue. Speak about your personal experiences. Do not explain or defend your position.

2. What is at the heart of the matter for you? Try to capture the essence of the matter and what is really important to you about this issue.

3. Within your overall experience, what are the gray areas? Describe those parts of the issue that feel unclear, uncertain, or fuzzy.

Resolution

Because there is a dearth of ethnic minority athletic trainers, it is important that you become a culturally competent and aware health care provider. This requires an understanding of delivery of health care to all individuals, not just with respect to race and ethnicity, but also sexual identity, sexual orientation, religion, class, and ability (physical and cognitive). It is also essential that you create an inclusive environment in which to treat athletes and patients and to attract prospective students to a career as a certified athletic trainer. Specific strategies might be to include diversity training as part of the orientation for new staff and students, create more opportunities for staff and student awareness and training in diversity issues, and adopt a broad statement on diversity that is prominent in your clinic and on your website. To create a pipeline for ethnic minority students and clinicians, you could hold high school health care profession workshops and career days for diverse populations and recruit ethnic minority students to athletic training on your own campus. Finally, you could become actively engaged in the work of the NATA's Ethnic Diversity Advisory Committee.

*Notes:*_____

_____

_____

_____

_____

_____

SCENARIO 22: TEAM PHYSICIAN CONFLICT WITH EMERGENCY MEDICAL SERVICE

My EMS agency provides a dedicated advanced life support ambulance for all varsity football games and, because the games frequently draw several thousand people, we also staff a second advanced life support unit for the spectators when possible. The dedicated unit is for the field, while the second unit may be pulled for calls in the community. As an athletic trainer and a paramedic, I am always assigned to the field unit and, for the game, I was working with an EMT partner who is well-known in the community. Just after the halftime band show, one of the majorettes came limping to our sideline location with severe foot pain. She was a family friend of the EMT and was crying to her "uncle" about her foot. We helped her into the ambulance, and my partner removed her shoe and started to evaluate her foot. It was clear that she had a metatarsal fracture, and he applied an ice pack while comforting her. My partner had known this patient since she was born because her father was a close friend. The patient calmed down and was resting comfortably on the stretcher when the team orthopedic surgeon suddenly appeared.

The surgeon jumped into the back of the ambulance, removed the ice pack, and started to palpate her foot. This caused the patient significant pain, and she started to cry again. My partner became irate and demanded to know what the surgeon was doing with his patient. I stood at the door of the ambulance and kept silent because I knew my partner could handle this situation. An argument ensued between my partner and the surgeon that became quite animated. Just as I thought I would have to intervene, a police officer came by and asked what was going on. The officer and my partner were also good friends, and my partner told the officer this doctor was interfering with his management of the patient. The surgeon said he was the team doctor and that we had to do what he said. The police officer reached into the ambulance, grabbed the doctor by his shirt, and pulled him out of the truck. The officer then told the doctor to go about his business or else he would be arrested for interfering with an EMS crew. The doctor was dumbfounded but left quietly.

Discussion Questions

1. Does a team doctor have a responsibility to care for injuries to students who are not players?

2. Should your EAP make provisions for injuries to band members, sideline photographers, or spectators?

3. Were the team doctor's actions appropriate considering that the patient was under the care of EMS and was resting comfortably prior to his arrival?

Resolution

My partner called the patient's father, who came to the ambulance. We applied a splint and helped the patient to her father's car, and he took her to a local hospital for x-rays. The police officer said he would file a report on the incident, and we also informed EMS management of the event. The doctor called the service manager on Monday and complained about our actions. The manager told the doctor he fully supported us and if he ever caused such a problem again, he would file a report with the local police chief, who also happened to be his father. Never underestimate the close relationship EMS has with community police departments. Although they may not always be as close as in this case, police officers will always side with EMS.

Additional Resolution

I would not have laughed out loud when the officer forcefully pulled the doctor out of the ambulance. That was unprofessional.

Notes:_____

_____

_____

_____

_____

SCENARIO 23: COMMUNICATING CARE
OUTSIDE OF THE UNIVERSITY SYSTEM

An athletic trainer in a dual appointment teaching and athletic training role with primary assignment to a collegiate baseball team in a somewhat rural area was experiencing difficulty in coordinating and monitoring the care of members of the baseball team. Over the course of the first baseball season she covered, many patients were seeking care outside of the university at the direction of their coach, who was a close friend of a physician assistant at an area clinic. The physician assistant had previously been certified as an athletic trainer but had let his licensure lapse without renewal and had a history of involvement with the university and the baseball program.

The team would not permit the female athletic trainer to travel, citing budgetary issues, but the physician assistant (who was male and funded his own way on road trips) attended a majority of the off-campus games and weekend road trips. At the end of the road trip, the athletic trainer would attempt to follow-up with the coach and the physician assistant regarding athlete status, any new injuries, or items of interest for the week. The coach and the physician assistant generalized issues and most often indicated that things were under control. On several occasions, the athletic trainer set treatment times, only to find out that many of the team members had already been to visit the physician assistant at the clinic earlier in the day and had received treatment. When the athletic trainer tried to follow-up with what care had been provided, the physician assistant would often not return telephone calls or e-mails or would not fully disclose what treatments had been provided to the patient. Documentation of all treatments was requested but not provided.

The athletic trainer reported and documented the lack of communication to the head athletic trainer and the athletic director. Meetings were held between the coach, athletic trainer, and head athletic trainer, but the physician assistant did not attend such meetings due to his busy schedule. The coach specifically indicated to the athletic trainer that if she or the university did anything to decrease the involvement of the physician assistant, he would quit his position as coach. Word of this statement was transferred to the athletic director, and the athletic trainer was instructed to try to more passively approach the situation.

At the end of the regular season, the team earned a spot in the playoffs, and travel to the regional tournament was organized. An invitation was extended to the athletic trainer to attend the tournament, which she accepted. The physician assistant also traveled to the tournament. While in the dugout, the team consistently sought out the physician assistant for care, and following the games each day, the athletic trainer was instructed that they were done for the day. She would schedule a treatment time for the athletes and when that time arrived, they would stop by to say they had already received treatment from the physician assistant.

Discussion Questions

1. What steps would you take early on to improve communication in a similar situation?

2. What potential legal issues are there for a university-affiliated athletic trainer when care is being sought off-campus and not communicated? What potential legal issues are there for a non–university-affiliated health care professional who is providing care to patients?

3. Discuss how the environment of an institution, including historical and geographical influences, might affect patient care. How might you be able to work to overcome barriers within a negative culture?

Resolution

Given the high level of competition and value of the athlete experience, the athletic trainer chose to remain passive during the tournament in order to not cause issues or undue stress to the athletes. The team ended up qualifying for the World Series. The athletic trainer followed up with the physician assistant to attain documentation from the treatments at the regional tournament, but she was unsuccessful. The athletic trainer evaluated the situation and determined the environment with the coach and physician assistant to be unpleasant and unproductive and sought the advice of the athletic director once more. The athletic director suggested the athletic trainer again be passive and not try to push the topic.

Given that the athletic trainer no longer believed she had a solid grasp on the overall team health and care being provided to them, she decided to inquire as to the possibility of turning over care and liability of the care to the physician assistant. The athletic director agreed that this was something that the school might support and would respond back. Ultimately, the athletic director agreed that the athletic trainer did not have to travel with the team to the World Series if she did not choose and that the physician assistant could provide care for the tournament.

Additional Resolution

There are multiple areas in which this scenario could have been changed or approached differently. Many historical components of the team and the athletic environment at this university played significantly into how it was handled from each representative. One specific point that could have been changed would have been to have the coach indicate the role of the physician assistant prior to the start of the season. Including him in more preseason items, rather than becoming quickly involved during the season, may have eased the tension. Perhaps even better would have been to indicate a clearly defined role on the sports medicine staff and affiliation with the university would have helped to clarify for the athletic trainer that his role was acceptable. In addition, although a line of communication was defined between the coach, athletic trainer, and physician assistant, it was not consistently followed. Having the support of administrators to remind these members of the communication practices would have been helpful.

*Notes:*_____

_____

_____

_____

Scenario 24: Language Barrier in the Athletic Training Facility

Oftentimes in professional sports, athletes from various countries and ethnic backgrounds collaborate to achieve a common goal. In professional baseball, athletes from all over the world compete in the United States. Many of these athletes speak different languages and dialects and often do not speak English very well. As an athletic trainer in this situation, it can be difficult to evaluate an injury, instruct athletes on proper form or technique, relay treatment or rehabilitation information, and educate athletes.

An athlete from the Dominican Republic entered the athletic training room and was clearly distressed. The athlete was drafted earlier in the month and had just arrived at the minor league affiliate where the athletic trainer had been working for the past few months. The athletic trainer did not speak Spanish (the athlete's first and only language) but could tell that something was wrong.

Discussion Questions

1. How can the athletic trainer communicate with the athlete in an accurate manner, ensuring his evaluation is precise and accurate?

2. Can the athletic trainer ask for help from anyone? Whom?

3. What legal principles or precedence must be considered?

Resolution

Prior to the season, the athletic trainer asked his supervisor how to approach this exact situation.

He was instructed to perform the following steps. Find someone on the coaching staff who was bilingual to assist in the evaluation of the injury and translation of rehabilitation directions. Make sure that the coach understands that he cannot talk about the player's injury or any medical information he may become privy to with anyone other than the medical staff. If possible, avoid using another player as an interpreter. Attempt to learn some basic phrases in Spanish (the second most popular language in baseball after English) such as, "Where does it hurt?" and "Are you ok?" Explain to the officials at the games that you do not speak Spanish and that if there is an injury on the field involving a Spanish-speaking athlete, you will need a coach to accompany you onto the field for evaluation purposes. When writing your SOAP (subjective, objective, assessment, and plan) notes, include that the evaluation or instructions were given through an interpreter and list that person as a reference.

The athletic trainer took the advice of the supervisor and used the bilingual pitching coach as his go-to interpreter for Spanish-speaking athletes. The coach was brought into the athletic training room, and the injury evaluation continued with no problems.

Additional Resolution

Because the coach was not formally trained in health care law or confidentiality, it would have been a good idea to have a more formal education session with the interpreter. Also, having the coach sign a disclosure form stating that he would not disclose any medical information would have been a good idea in this situation.

Editor's Note

Hospitals have strict rules regarding the use of interpreters, and these rules are based on guidelines issued by the federal government. Use of family or friends to interpret during emergencies may be the only alternative at times, but these resources should never be used as a frontline means to overcome language barriers. Telecommunication services are available for any language from professional language organizations. I have been deployed to international disasters, and the value of competent translators is invaluable, but learning a few words of the native language can make a very sick patient feel at ease.

Notes:_____

_____

_____

SCENARIO 25: CIRCUMVENTION OF POLICY

An athletic trainer was working with the track and field team at a large university. One of the coaches for the team was a strong believer in chiropractic care for low back pain. The athletic department did not have a chiropractor on staff, although a relationship had been established with one of the chiropractors in the community for referral of athletes when deemed appropriate by a team physician. The coach in question had expressed his preference for a different chiropractor and had also questioned why it was necessary for an athlete to first be seen by a team physician prior to a referral being made to any outside provider. On at least one prior occasion, the coach had directed an athlete to go directly to the chiropractor he preferred without notifying the athletic trainer or the team physician about the back pain problem. You had discussed with the coach the reasons for the policy being in place and asked him to not circumvent the policy in the future. One day, one of the track athletes went to see the athletic trainer, complaining of worsening low back pain. She said the pain started several weeks ago and the coach told her to go see the chiropractor he preferred without first notifying the athletic trainer or the team physician. She had been treated several times by the chiropractor, but her pain had only gotten worse.

Discussion Questions

1. What should the primary initial concern of the athletic trainer be in this case?

2. What are some of the likely reasons behind the department policy that an athlete must first be seen by a team physician before an outside referral can be made?

3. What are some possibilities for how the athletic trainer could handle approaching this coach for further discussion about this issue?

Resolution

Work-up of the athlete revealed she had a stress fracture in one of her lumbar vertebrae. Her activity was modified, and she began a formal rehabilitation program. A meeting was called involving the coach in question, the head coach, the head athletic trainer, and the team physician. The policy was again explained, as well as the reasons for the way it is structured. The current case served as an excellent illustration of why the policy was in place, and the coach in question seemed to have a good understanding of the risks of circumventing the policy. He agreed not to do so in the future.

Notes:_____

_____

_____

_____

_____

_____

II

APPENDICES

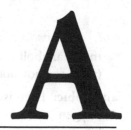

Glossary of
Sports Medicine Terms

A

abdomen: The part of the body that contains the stomach, small intestine, colon, rectum, liver, spleen, pancreas, kidneys, appendix, gallbladder, and bladder.

abduct: Movement of any extremity away from the midline of the body. This action is achieved by an abductor muscle.

abrasion: Any injury that rubs off the surface of the skin.

abscess: An infection that produces pus; can be the result of a blister, callus, penetrating wound, or laceration.

Achilles tendon: One of the longest tendons in the body; it attaches the calf muscles to the heel bone.

acromioclavicular (AC) joint: Joint of the shoulder where the acromion process of the scapula and the distal end of the clavicle meet; most shoulder separations occur at this point.

acute: Sudden, brief, and severe; usually referred to in connection with a new illness or injury.

adduct: Movement of an extremity toward the midline of the body. This action is achieved by an adductor muscle.

adhesion: Abnormal adherence of collagen fibers to surrounding structures during immobilization following trauma or as a complication of surgery that restricts normal elasticity of the structures involved.

advanced life support (ALS): Advanced medical care, including intravenous access, defibrillation, advanced airway interventions, and medication administration.

aerobic: Exercise in which energy needed is supplied by oxygen inspired and is required for sustained periods of vigorous exercise with a continually high pulse rate.

anabolic steroids: Steroids that promote tissue growth by creating protein in an attempt to enhance muscle growth; the

Gorse KM, Feld F, Blanc RO, eds.
Athletic Training Case Scenarios:
Domain-Based Situations and Solutions (pp 227-242).
© 2016 Taylor & Francis Group.

main anabolic steroid is testosterone (male sex hormone).

anaerobic: Exercise without the use of oxygen as an energy source; short bursts of vigorous exercise.

anaphylactic shock: Shock that is caused by an allergic reaction.

anaphylaxis: Severe allergic response to a substance. Symptoms include wheezing, itching, nasal congestion, hives, immediate intense burning of hands and feet, collapse with severe drop in blood pressure, loss of consciousness, and cardiac arrest.

anatomy: The study of the structure and parts of the body.

androgen: A hormone, such as testosterone, responsible for the development of male characteristics.

anterior: In front of; the front surface of.

anterior compartment syndrome: Condition in which swelling within the anterior compartment of the lower leg jeopardizes the viability of muscles, nerves, and arteries that serve the foot. In severe cases, emergency surgery is necessary to relieve the swelling and pressure.

anterior cruciate ligament (ACL): A primary stabilizing ligament within the center of the knee joint that prevents hyperextension and excessive rotation of the joint. A complete tear of the ACL necessitating reconstruction could require up to 12 months of rehabilitation.

anterior talofibular ligament: A ligament of the ankle that connects the fibula (lateral ankle bone) to the talus. This ligament is often subject to sprain.

anti-inflammatory: Any agent that prevents inflammation, such as aspirin or ibuprofen.

arteriogram: A film demonstrating arteries after the injection of a dye.

arthrogram: X-ray technique for joints using air and/or dye injected into the affected area; useful in diagnosing meniscus tears of the knee and rotator cuff tears of the shoulder.

arthroscope: An instrument used in surgery to visualize the interior of a joint cavity.

arthroscopy: A surgical examination of the internal structures of a joint by means of viewing through an arthroscope. An arthroscopic procedure can be used to remove or repair damaged tissue or as a diagnostic procedure to inspect the extent of any damage or confirm a diagnosis.

aspiration: The withdrawal of fluid from a body cavity by means of a suction or a siphonage apparatus, such as a syringe.

asymptomatic: Without symptoms.

athletic trainer: One who has certification from the National Athletic Trainers' Association (NATA).

atrophy: To shrivel or shrink from disuse, as in muscular atrophy.

avascular necrosis: Death of a body part due to lack of circulation.

avulsion: The forcible tearing away of a part or structure.

B

Baker's cyst: Localized swelling of a bursa sac in the posterior knee as a result of fluid that has escaped from the knee capsule; indicates that there is a trauma inside the knee joint that leads to excessive fluid production.

basic life support (BLS): Basic medical care provided by emergency medical technicians.

Bennett's fracture: A fracture and dislocation of the base of the first metacarpal (the thumb).

blowout fracture: A fracture of the cavity containing the eyeball and its associated muscles that can be the result of a direct blow to the eye or cheek.

bone scan: An imaging procedure in which a radioactive-labeled substance is injected into the body to determine the status of a bony injury. If the radioactive substance is taken up by the bone at the injury site, the injury will show as a hot spot on the scan image. The bone scan is particularly useful in the diagnosis of stress fractures.

brachial plexus: Network of nerves originating from the cervical vertebrae and running down to the shoulder, arm, hand, and fingers.

bruise: A discoloration of the skin due to an extravasation of blood into the underlying tissues.

bursa: A fluid-filled sac that is located in areas where friction is likely to occur, then minimizes the friction (eg, between a tendon and a bone).

C

calcaneofibular ligament: The ligament that connects the fibula to the calcaneus.

calf: Large muscle located at the back of the shin that includes the gastrocnemius and the soleus muscles and is connected to the heel by the Achilles tendon; responsible for foot plantarflexion and instrumental in jumping.

capsule: An enclosing structure that surrounds the joint and contains ligaments that stabilize that joint.

cardiopulmonary resuscitation (CPR): Combined artificial ventilation and cardiac massage technique for reviving a person whose heart and breathing have stopped and who is unconscious.

cartilage: Smooth, slippery substance preventing 2 ends of bones from rubbing together and grating.

cellulitis: Inflammation of cellular or connective tissue.

cervical vertebrae: Group of 7 vertebrae located in the neck.

chondromalacia: Roughening of the articular cartilage. Best known for the roughening of the underside of the patella, which can occur in any patellofemoral injury.

chronic: Of long duration, often years; recurring; opposite of acute.

clavicle: The collar bone.

coccyx: The tail bone; a group of 4 vertebrae that are fused together, located at the terminal end of the spine.

cold pack: A pack of natural or synthetic ice that is applied to any injury to minimize blood flow in the area to control the injury.

collagen substance: Exists in commonly injured tissues of the body, including skin, cartilage, ligaments, and bone.

collateral ligament: On either side of, and acting as a radius of movement of, a hinge joint, such as of the elbow, knee and wrist.

Colles fracture: A fracture of the distal end of the radius, with the lower end being displaced backward.

compartment syndrome: A build-up of pressure in muscles.

complex carbohydrate: A substance that contains several sugar units linked together, such as starch.

computed tomography (CT): Method of visualizing the body's soft tissues. Using x-rays with the beam passing repeatedly through the body part, the CT scans while a computer calculates tissue absorption at each point scanned.

computed tomography (CT) scan: An imaging technique that uses a computer to organize the information from multiple radiograph views and construct a cross-sectional image of areas inside the body. Also known as *computerized axial tomography (CAT)* or *CT scan.*

concentric muscle contraction: A shortening of the muscle as it develops tension and contracts to move a resistance.

concussion: Jarring injury of the brain. It can be graded as mild, moderate, or severe depending on loss of consciousness, amnesia, and loss of equilibrium.

congenital: Existing before birth; to be born with.

conjunctivitis: Inflammation of the membrane lining the eyelids and covering the eyeball.

connective tissue: A material consisting of fibers that form a framework that provides support structure for body tissues.

continuous passive motion (CPM): Constant passive motion devices used in the early stage of knee rehabilitation.

contract: To shorten a muscle body.

contractures: Abnormal, usually permanent, contraction of a muscle due to atrophy of muscle fibers, extensive scar tissue over a joint, or other factors.

contusion: An injury to a muscle and tissues caused by a blow from a blunt object, typically resulting in a bruise.

coronary artery disease: Narrowing or blockage of one or more of the coronary arteries, resulting in decreased blood supply to the heart (ischemia). Also known as *ischemic heart disease.*

coronary disease: Damage to the heart when insufficient blood flows through the vessels because they are blocked with fat or have become thick and hard; this harms the muscles of the heart.

cortical steroids: Used to suppress joint inflammation.

cortisol: The major natural glucocorticoid in humans; the primary stress hormone.

cortisone: A steroid hormone that is used to treat many autoimmune or inflammatory diseases, including rheumatoid arthritis.

costochondral: Cartilage that separates the bones within the rib cage.

cramp: A painful, involuntary, spasmodic contraction.

cranium: Bony framework of the skull, consisting of 8 cranial bones, 14 bones of the face, and the teeth.

cryotherapy: A treatment (modality) with use of cold.

D

debridement: Removal of nonhealthy tissues and foreign material from a wound or burn to prevent infection and permit healing.

defibrillator: Machine used to deliver an electrical shock to the chest to stop ventricular fibrillation; it may be internal (implanted) or external.

degenerative disk disease: The pathological process by which an intervertebral disk becomes progressively disrupted and fails in its functions.

degenerative joint disease: Changes in the joint surfaces as a result of repetitive trauma.

dehydration: A lack of an adequate amount of fluid in the body; may be accompanied by dry mouth, thirst, constipation, concentrated urine, or fever. Dehydration occurs when a person's body water content has decreased to a dangerously low level. Water accounts for 60% of a man's weight and 50% of a woman's weight.

deltoid ligament: Ligament that connects the tibia to bones of the medial aspect of the foot and is primarily responsible for stability of the ankle on the medial side.

deltoid muscle: Muscles at the top of the arm, just below the shoulder; responsible for shoulder motions to the front, side, and back.

diagnosis: Identification of a disease or disorder by a physician.

diaphragm muscle: The thin, muscular partition below the lungs and heart that separates the chest cavity from the abdominal cavity.

diastole: Period during the heart cycle in which the muscle relaxes, followed by contraction (systole). In a blood pressure reading, the lower number is the diastolic measurement.

diastolic blood pressure: The pressure of the blood in the main arteries, which rises and falls as the muscles of the body cope with varying demands (eg, exercise, stress, sleep). Two types of

pressures are measured: (1) systolic pressure, created by the contraction of the heart muscle pushing blood into the vessels and (2) diastolic pressure, when the heart is at rest between beats. A reading of 120/80 is said to be the normal range. Blood pressure that is too high (hypertension) can cause health problems, such as heart attacks and strokes.

dilate: To expand or open a structure, such as the pupil of the eye or a passageway, such as an artery.

dilated: Enlarged (as in pupils).

disk, intervertebral: A flat, rounded plate between each vertebrae of the spine. The disk consists of a thick fiber ring, which surrounds a soft gel-like interior. It functions as a cushion and shock absorber for the spinal column.

dislocation: Complete displacement of joint surfaces.

distal: Term referencing one anatomical term away from another; for example, the hand is distal to the elbow.

dorsiflexion: Ankle motion, such that the foot and toes are moved away from the ground in an upward fashion.

dorsum: The back; the back surface of any part.

dysfunction: Unable to function normally as a body organ or system.

E

eccentric muscle contraction: An overall lengthening of the muscle as it develops tension and contracts to control motion performed by an outside force; often referred to as a negative contraction in weight training.

ecchymosis: Bleeding into the surface tissue below the skin, resulting in a black and blue effect.

edema: Accumulation of fluid in organs and tissues of the body; swelling.

efferent: Away from, pushing toward the center.

effusion: Accumulation of fluid, or the fluid itself, in various spaces in the body. Commonly, the knee has an effusion after an injury.

electrical galvanic stimulation (EGS): An electrical therapeutic modality that sends a current to the body at select voltages and frequencies to stimulate pain receptors, disperse edema, or neutralize muscle spasms, among other functional applications.

electrolyte: Ionized salts in blood, tissue fluids, and cells, including salts of sodium, potassium, and chlorine.

electromyogram (EMG): Test to determine nerve function.

emergency medical service (EMS): System in communities that delivers prehospital care to the sick and injured.

emergency medical technician (EMT): Ambulance personnel that have completed a minimum of 120 hours of training and are capable of delivering basic life support care, including oxygen administration, splinting, vital signs, and physical examination.

epicondylitis: Inflammation in the elbow due to overuse.

etiology: Study of the causes of injury and disease.

eversion: Action of the ankle turning outward.

extension: Action of straightening of a joint as achieved by an extensor muscle.

external rotation: Lateral movement of a joint or extremity to the outside.

F

fascia: A connective tissue sheath consisting of fibrous tissue and fat, which unites the skin to the underlying tissue.

fasting blood glucose test: A diagnostic test for diabetes mellitus that is performed at a laboratory or doctor's office. The procedure involves testing a blood sample, which is usually taken in the morning before eating, for glucose. A level greater than 140 mg/dL is generally considered diagnostic for diabetes mellitus.

fat percentage: The amount of body weight that is adipose, fat tissue. Fat percentages can be calculated by underwater weighing, measuring select skin fold thickness, or by analyzing electrical impedance.

femur: Thigh bone; the longest bone in the body.

fibula: Smaller of the 2 bones in the lower leg; runs from the knee to the ankle along the outside of the lower leg.

flexibility exercise: General term used to describe exercise performed by a player to passively or actively elongate soft tissue without the assistance of an athletic trainer.

flexion: Motion of bending a joint as achieved by a flexor muscle.

fracture: Breach in continuity of a bone. Types of fractures include simple, compound, comminuted, greenstick, incomplete, impacted, longitudinal, oblique, stress, and transverse.

frostbite: Damage to the tissues from exposure to temperatures below 32°F (0°C). An initial pins-and-needles sensation is followed by numbness. After that, the skin appears white, cold, and hard and finally becomes red and swollen.

·G

gamekeeper's thumb: Tear of the ulnar collateral ligament of the metacarpophalangeal joint of the thumb.

glenohumeral: The shoulder girdle; consists of the glenoid capsule, head of the humerus, and labrum; the type of joint that allows 360-degree motion (a ball and socket joint).

glenoid: Cavity of the scapula into which the head of the humerus fits to form the shoulder girdle.

glucose: A simple sugar found in the blood; all carbohydrates and some fats can be changed into glucose by the body. It is the body's main source of energy. Also known as *dextrose*.

glycogen: Stored form of carbohydrate in the liver and muscles. Glycogen is the chief source of stored fuel in the body.

grade one injury (first degree): A mild injury in which a ligament, tendon, or other musculoskeletal tissue may have been stretched or contused but not torn or otherwise disrupted.

grade three injury (third degree): A severe injury in which the tissue has been significantly, and in some cases totally, torn or has been otherwise disrupted, causing a virtual total loss of function.

grade two injury (second degree): A moderate injury in which the musculoskeletal tissue has been partially, but not totally, torn, which causes appreciable limitation in function of the injured tissue.

groin: Junction of the thigh and abdomen; location of the muscles that rotate, flex, and adduct the hip.

guarding: Involuntary local reflex (protective) abdominal muscle contraction in the region of an area of peritonitis (inflamed lining membrane of the potential cavity in the abdomen).

H

hammer toe: Condition in which the first digit of a toe is at a different angle than the remaining digits of the same toe.

hamstring: Category of muscle that runs from the buttocks to the knee along the back of the thigh. It functions to flex the knee and is often injured as a result of improper conditioning or lack of muscle flexibility.

heat cramps: Painful muscle spasms of the arms or legs caused by excessive body heat and depletion of fluids and electrolytes.

heat exhaustion: Mild form of shock due to dehydration because of excessive sweating when exposed to heat and humidity.

heat stroke: Condition of rapidly rising internal body temperature that overwhelms the body's mechanisms for release of heat and could result in death if not cared for appropriately.

heel cup: Orthotic device that is inserted into the shoe and worn under the heel to give support to the Achilles tendon and help absorb impacts at the heel.

helicopter emergency medical services (HEMS): Helicopter service capable of landing in the field to evacuate critically injured or ill patients and transporting them to a trauma center or higher-level hospital; usually staffed by a combination of flight nurses, flight paramedics, or physicians. Also known as *air medical evacuation*, these helicopters carry blood and have advanced medications and skills that are not commonly found on ground ambulances. Helicopters are also used to transfer patients from small hospitals to tertiary care hospitals.

hemarthrosis: Accumulation of blood within a joint as a result of an acute injury.

hematoma: Tumor-like mass produced by an accumulation of coagulated blood in a cavity.

hemorrhage: To bleed.

herniate: To protrude through an abnormal body opening.

high-density lipoprotein (HDL) cholesterol: A type of cholesterol thought to help protect against atherosclerosis; good cholesterol.

hip pointer: Contusion to the iliac crest.

hot pack: Chemical pack that rests in water, is approximately 160°F, and retains its heat for 15 to 20 minutes when placed in a towel for general therapeutic application.

humerus: Bone of the upper arm that runs from the shoulder to the elbow.

hyaline cartilage: Most common type of cartilage.

hydrotherapy: Treatment (modality) using water.

hyperextension: Extreme or over extension of a limb or body part.

I

ice massage: Ice formed into a device, such as a paper cup, that is rubbed on an injury in a massaging action to achieve a level of numbness.

iliac crest: Lateral edge of the hip; generally the site of a hip pointer.

iliotibial band: A thick, wide muscle layer that runs from the iliac crest to the knee joint and is occasionally inflamed as a result of excessive running.

impingement syndrome: Pinching together of the supraspinatus muscle and other soft tissue in the shoulder. The most common (throwing) arm injury, which represents many pathologies and generally involves supraspinatus overuse.

inferior: Anatomically beneath, lower, or toward the bottom.

inflammation: The body's natural response to injury in which the injury site might display various degrees of pain, swelling, heat, redness, and/or loss of function.

intermittent compression pump: Therapeutic modality that uses an air pump to send air into a sleeve worn over an injury, on an intermittent basis, to disperse edema and break up swelling at the injury.

internal rotation: Rotation of a joint of an extremity medially, to the inside.

interosseous membrane: Uniting membrane between the tibia and fibula that forms a collagenous fibrous tissue. It has 2 functions: to serve as an origin for many of the muscles of the lower leg and to transmit stress from the tibia to the fibula.

intrinsic: Inherent or inside.

intubation: Use of a laryngoscope to place a breathing tube into the trachea. Also known as *endotracheal intubation (ETI)*, it is a skill reserved for physicians, nurse anesthetists, flight nurses, paramedics, and respiratory therapists in some areas of the country.

isokinetic exercise: Form of active resistive exercise in which the speed of limb movement is controlled by a preset limiting exercise machine.

isometric contraction: Muscular contraction in which tension is developed but no mechanical work is done. There is no appreciable joint movement, and the overall length of the muscle stays the same.

isotonic contraction: A concentric or eccentric muscular contraction that results in the movement of a joint or body part, as in lifting a weight.

J

joint: The point of juncture between 2 or more bones where movement occurs.

joint mobilization: Passive traction and/ or gliding movements applied to joint surfaces that maintain or restore the joint play normally allowed by the capsule so that the normal roll-slide joint mechanisms can occur as the player moves.

K

ketone: A breakdown product of fat that accumulates in the blood as a result of inadequate insulin or inadequate calorie intake.

ketosis: A condition of having ketone bodies build up in body tissues and fluids. The signs of ketosis are nausea, vomiting, and stomach pain.

kyphosis: Excessive curvature of the upper spine, resulting in humpback, hunchback, or rounding of the shoulders.

L

labrum (labrum glenoid): The cartilage of the glenoid cavity in the shoulder.

lateral: To the outside of the body.

lateral collateral ligament (LCL): Ligament of the knee along the lateral aspect that connects the femur to the fibula. It provides lateral stability to the joint.

left ventricle: The largest and most muscular chamber of the heart concerned with the pumping of oxygen-rich blood from the lungs (via the left atrium) to all the other tissues of the body, via the aorta.

lesion: Wound, injury, or tumor.

ligament: Band of fibrous tissue that connects bone to bone or bone to cartilage and supports and strengthens joints.

lipid: Descriptive term for a fat or fat-like substance found in the blood, such as cholesterol. The body stores fat as energy for future use, just like a car that has a reserve fuel tank. When the body needs energy, it can break down the lipids into fatty acids and burn them like glucose (sugar).

low-density lipoprotein (LDL) cholesterol: This cholesterol provides for necessary body functions, but in excessive amounts, it tends to accumulate in artery walls; also known as *bad cholesterol.*

lumbar vertebrae: Five vertebrae of the lower back that articulate with the sacrum to form the lumbosacral joint.

lumbosacral: Region of low back that comprises the lumbar and sacral spine.

lungs: The 2 organs of respiration that bring air and blood into close contact so that oxygen can be added to and carbon dioxide can be removed from the blood.

lymphatic system: The tissues and organs that produce, store, and carry cells that fight infection. This system includes the bone marrow, spleen, thymus, lymph nodes, and vessels that carry lymph.

M

magnetic resonance imaging (MRI): Imaging procedure in which a radio frequency pulse causes certain electrical elements of the injured tissue to react to this pulse; through this process, a computer display and permanent film establish a visual image. MRI does not require radiation and is useful in the diagnosis of soft tissue, disk, and meniscus injuries.

malleolus: Rounded projection on either side of the ankle joint; the lateral malleolus is the fibula and the medial malleolus is the tibia.

mallet finger: Injury of the fingertip in which the extension tendon is avulsed off the distal phalanx.

manipulation: A passive movement using physiological or accessory motion, which may be applied with a thrust or when the player is under anesthesia.

maximal aerobic power (MAX VO$_2$): The maximal volume of oxygen consumed per unit of time.

medial: To the inside of the body.

medial collateral ligament (MCL): Ligament of the knee along the medial aspect that connects the femur to the joint.

meniscectomy: An intra-articular surgical procedure of the knee by which all or part of the damaged meniscus is removed.

meniscus: Crescent-shaped cartilage, usually pertaining to the knee joint; also known as *cartilage.* There are 2 menisci in the knee: medial and lateral. They work to absorb weight within the knee and provide stability.

metacarpals: Five long bones of the hand, running from the wrist to the fingers.

metatarsals: Five long bones of the foot, running from the ankle to the toes.

Morton's neuroma: Involves the nerves and is usually the result of a trauma to the foot, causing inflammation and sharp pain, usually between the third and fourth toes.

Morton's toe: A hereditary condition in which the second toe is longer than the first toe. This can cause mechanical imbalances that produce pain with weightbearing.

muscle: Body tissues that consist of cells that contract when lengthened or straightened.

myositis: Inflammation of a muscle.

myositis ossificans traumatica: A benign ossification, usually following severe trauma to a large muscle.

N

National Athletic Trainers' Association (NATA): The governing body of the athletic training profession.

necrotic: Relating to the death of a portion of tissue.

neoprene: Lightweight rubber used in joint and muscle sleeves designed to provide support and/or insulation to the area.

nerve: One or more fibers or bundles of fibers that form a part of a system in the body that conveys impulses of sensation, motion, etc, between the spinal cord or brain and other body parts.

neuritis: Inflammation of a nerve.

neurologist: A doctor who specializes in the diagnosis and treatment of disorders of the nervous system.

neuromuscular: Pertaining to the nerves and muscles.

neuron: A nerve cell.

neuropathy: Group of symptoms caused by abnormalities in sensory or motor nerves. Symptoms include tingling and numbness in the hands or feet, followed by gradually progressive muscular weakness. The 3 major forms of nerve damage are peripheral neuropathy, autonomic neuropathy, and mononeuropathy. The most common form is peripheral neuropathy, which mainly affects the feet and legs.

neurotransmitter: Chemicals that act as messengers between cells in the brain and nervous system that transmit impulses across the gap from a neuron to another neuron, a muscle, or a gland.

O

obesity: Obesity occurs when a person has too much body fat. Obesity is not the same as being overweight; a person is considered obese when they weigh 20% or more of the maximum desirable weight for their height.

olecranon process: Bony projection of the ulna at the tip of the elbow.

one repetition maximum: The maximum amount of weight that can be lifted by the player in a particular exercise at one time. This is used as a strength testing technique.

orthotic: Any device applied to or around the body in the care of physical impairment or disability, commonly used to control foot mechanics.

osteochondritis dissecans: A piece of bone and/or cartilage loosened from its attachment after trauma and a cause of a lesion.

osteomyelitis: An inflammatory disease of bone caused usually by infection with *Streptococcus* or *Staphylococcus*.

osteoporosis: Loss of calcium and other substances from bones, causing bones to become weak and prone to fractures.

overuse syndromes: A result of repetitive stress to body structures.

oxidation: Combining a substance with oxygen.

P

paramedic: Ambulance personnel that have completed more than 1000 hours of training and deliver advanced life support care.

paresthesia: Sensation of numbness or tingling, indicating nerve irritation.

patella: The kneecap. The patella functions to protect the distal end of the femur as well as increase the mechanical advantage and force-generating capacities of the quadriceps muscle group.

patella tendinitis: Inflammation of the patellar ligament. Also known as *jumper's knee.*

patellofemoral joint: Articulation of the kneecap and femur. Inflammation of this joint can occur through (1) acute injury to the patella; (2) overuse from excessive running, particularly if there is an associated knee weakness; (3) chronic wear and tear of the knee; and (4) as a result of poor foot mechanics. Patellofemoral irritation can lead to chondromalacia, which in its most chronic condition, could require surgery.

pathology: Study of the nature and cause of injury.

pectorals: Chest muscles beneath the breast that lead up to the shoulder.

peroneal muscles: Group of muscles of the lateral lower leg that are responsible for eversion of the ankle. Tendons of these 3 muscles are vital to the stability of the ankle and foot.

phalanx: Any bone of the fingers or toes; plural is *phalanges.*

phlebitis: Inflammation of a vein.

phonophoresis: The technique of driving whole molecules of medication with ultrasound.

plantar: Pertaining to the sole of the foot.

plantar fascia: The tight band of muscle beneath the arch of the foot.

plantar fasciitis: Inflammation of the plantar fascia; associated with overuse or acute foot injury.

plantarflexion: Ankle motion such that the toes are pointed toward the ground.

plica: Fold of tissue in the joint capsule and a common result of knee injury.

posterior: At the back part, or rear, of the body.

posterior cruciate ligament (PCL): A primary stabilizing ligament of the knee that provides significant stability and prevents displacement of the tibia backward within the knee joint. A complete tear of this ligament necessitating reconstruction could require up to 12 months of rehabilitation.

Professional Baseball Athletic Trainers Society (PBATS): The governing body of athletic trainers in professional baseball.

progressive resistance exercise (PRE): An approach to exercise whereby the load or resistance to the muscle is applied by some mechanical means and is quantitatively and progressively increased over time.

pronation: In the foot, it is a combination of motions resulting in a position such that the foot is placed in abduction and eversion. In the hand, pronation is the movement of the forearm into a palm-down position.

proprioceptive neuromuscular facilitation: An approach to therapeutic exercise based on the principles of functional human anatomy and neurophysiology.

proximal: Near the source, nearest any point being described.

Q

Q-angle: Normal angle of the quadriceps relative to the patella. The normal angle for males is 10 degrees.

quadriceps: Also known as *quads*; a group of muscles of the front thigh that run from the hip and form a common tendon at the patella that are responsible for knee extension.

R

radial pulse: Pulse felt at the wrist.

radiate: Pain that seems to travel from one point in the musculature to another.

radiography: Taking of x-rays.

radius: Forearm bone on the thumb side.

Raynaud's phenomenon: Changes in skin color due to spasm of small blood vessels, especially with exposure to cold.

recommended dietary allowance: In the United States, the amount of an essential nutrient that is recommended on a daily basis to maintain health in various age groups and categories, as determined by a board of nutrition experts; used in labeling of foods.

reconstruction: Surgical rebuilding of a joint using natural, artificial, or transplanted materials.

referred pain: Pain felt in an undamaged area of the body away from the actual injury.

reflex (deep tendon): Contraction of a muscle in response to tapping the tendon or guider with a reflex hammer; it requires intact sensory nerve supply to transmit the stretching of receptors in the muscle and intact motor nerve supply for the muscle to contract.

resect: To cut off, or cut out, a portion of a structure or organ.

retraction: The moving of tissue to expose a part or structure of the body.

risk factor: A factor that increases the chance of developing or aggravating a condition.

rotator cuff: Comprises 4 muscles in the shoulder area, including the supraspinatus (most commonly injured), infraspinatus, teres minor, and subscapularis, that can be irritated by overuse.

rotator cuff impingement syndrome: A microtrauma or overuse injury caused by stress. The 4 stages are (1) tendentious with temporary thickening of the bursa and rotator cuff, (2) fiber dissociation in the tendon with permanent thickening of the bursa and scar formation, (3) a partial rotator cuff tear of less than 1 cm, and (4) a complete tear of 1 cm or more.

S

sacroiliac: Junction of the sacrum with the hip bone.

sacrum: Group of 5 fused vertebrae located just below the lumbar vertebrae of the low back.

scapula: Shoulder blade.

sciatic nerve: Major nerve that carries impulses for muscular action and sensations between the low back and thigh and lower leg; it is the longest nerve in the body.

sciatica: Irritation of the sciatic nerve, resulting in pain or tingling running down the inside of the leg.

shin splint: A catch-all syndrome describing pain in the shin that is not a fracture or tumor and cannot be defined otherwise.

shock: Inadequate tissue perfusion of vital organs, such as the brain, heart, and kidneys. Early signs are an altered level of consciousness, rapid heart rate, increased respiratory rate, pale skin, diaphoresis, and, ultimately, systemic collapse. Hypotension is a late sign of shock. Untreated shock will result in cardiac arrest.

spasm: Muscle soreness induced by exercise; it is the result of reduced muscle blood flow, which results in pain.

spinous process: A small projection off the posterior portion of each vertebra that functions as an attachment site for muscles or ligaments of the spine.

spleen: Large solid organ responsible for the normal production and destruction of blood cells.

spondylitis: Inflammation of one or more vertebrae.

spondylolisthesis: Forward displacement of one vertebra over another below it due to a developmental defect in the vertebrae.

spondylosis: Abnormal vertebral fixation or immobility.

sports psychology: A science that deals with the mental and emotional aspects of physical performance.

sprain: Injury resulting from the stretch or twist of the joint that causes various degrees of stretch or tear of a ligament or other soft tissue at the joint.

sternoclavicular (SC) joint: Articulation of the collarbone with the sternum.

sternum: The breast bone.

steroids: Any one of several hormone-like substances. *See anabolic steroids* and *cortical steroids.*

strain: Injury resulting from a pull or torsion to the muscle or tendon that causes various degrees of stretch or tear to the muscle or tendon tissue.

stress fracture: A hairline type of break in a bone caused by overuse.

stress x-ray: A continual x-ray taken when a portion of the body is stressed to its maximum to determine joint stability. This test is used in some ankle injuries.

stretching: Any therapeutic maneuver designed to elongate shortened soft tissue structures and thereby increase flexibility.

subluxation: Partial dislocation of a joint. The term usually implies that the joint can return to its normal position without formal reduction.

superior: In anatomy, the upper of 2 parts; toward the top or above.

supination: Movement of the forearm into a palm-up position.

synovial fluid: Lubricating fluid for joints and tendons, produced in synovium, or the inner lining of a joint.

synovitis: Inflammation of the synovial lining of a joint.

systole: The portion of the heart cycle during which the heart muscle is contracting.

systolic blood pressure: The highest blood pressure produced by the contraction of the heart. Recorded as the first number in your blood pressure measurement.

T

talus: The ankle bone that articulates with the tibia and fibula to form the ankle joint.

target heart rate: A predetermined pulse to be obtained during exercise when circulation is working at full efficient capacities.

tarsals: Group of 6 bones of the foot, including the navicular, talus, cuboid, and 3 cuneiform bones.

temporomandibular joint (TMJ): The articulation of the jaw and skull; considered by some to be vital in resolution of injuries throughout the body.

tendinitis: Inflammation of the tendon and/or tendon sheath caused by chronic overuse or sudden injury.

tendon: Tissue that connects muscle to bone.

tennis elbow: General term for lateral elbow pain.

thermotherapy: Use of heat to treat a disease or disorder.

thoracic: Group of 12 vertebrae located in the thorax; it articulates with the 12 ribs.

thoracic outlet compression syndrome: A neurovascular disorder of the upper extremity that is common in throwing.

tibia: Larger of the 2 bones of the lower leg that is the weightbearing bone of the shin.

tomograph: A special type of x-ray apparatus that demonstrates an organ or tissue at a particular depth.

trachea: The windpipe.

transcutaneous electrical nerve stimulator (TENS): An electrical modality that sends a mild current though pads at the injury site, which stimulates the brain to release the natural analgesic, endorphin.

transverse process: Small lateral projection off the right and left side of each vertebrae that functions as an attachment site for muscles and ligaments of the spine.

trapezius: Flat, triangular muscle covering the posterior surface of the neck and shoulder.

triangular cartilage: A connective tissue characterized by its nonvascularity and firm consistency; located on the little finger side of the wrist.

triceps: Muscle of the back of the upper arm that is primarily responsible for extending the elbow.

U

ulna: Forearm bone that runs from the tip of the elbow to the little finger side of the wrist.

ulnar collateral ligament: A band or sheet of fibrous tissue connecting 2 or more bones, cartilages, or other structures or serving as support for fasciae or muscles; located on the inside of the elbow. (Ligament that was replaced or repaired for the Tommy John surgery.)

ulnar nerve: Nerve in the elbow commonly irritated from excessive throwing.

ultrasound: An electrical modality that transmits a sound wave through an applicator into the skin to the soft tissue to heat the local area for relaxing the injured tissue and/or disperse edema.

unconscious: An impairment of brain function in which the individual is not conscious and is unable to respond to sensory stimuli.

V

valgus: Angulation outward and away from the midline of the body.

varus: Angulation inward and toward the midline of the body.

vasoconstriction: Decrease of local blood flow.

vital signs: Respiration, heart rate, and body temperature.

vitamin: Any of the many organic substances that are vital in small amounts to the normal functioning of the body. Vitamins are found in food, produced by the body, and manufactured synthetically; along with minerals, they are known as *micronutrients*.

W

wheezing: A whistling noise in the chest that occurs during breathing when the airways are compressed.

whirlpool: Water bath in which the water is propelled by air to produce a massaging therapeutic action.

wind knocked out: Syndrome describing a contraction of the abdominal nerve trunk, the solar plexus, as a result of an abdominal contusion.

wrist: The junction between the 2 forearm bones (radius and ulna) and the 8 wrist bones (trapezium, trapezoid, capitate, hamate, pisiform, triquetral, lunate, and scaphoid).

Y

yield point: The maximum load that a material can sustain without permanent deformation.

Z

zygoma: The cheekbone.

B

Athletic Training
Terminology

The Mission Statement for the National Athletic Trainers' Association (NATA) (www.nata.org) is:

The mission of the National Athletic Trainers' Association is to enhance the quality of health care provided by certified athletic trainers and to advance the athletic training profession.

USE OF "ATC"

Communication among athletic training professionals and from athletic trainers to external audiences is extremely important. Members often ask about the use of *ATC* and other terms. NATA's policy is not to use the ATC acronym as a noun; ATC is an acronym that describes a credential, not a person, and it should only be used following the name of a certified individual. Using the ATC acronym as a noun inhibits the Board of Certification's ability to protect the ATC credential against misuse. In other words, NATA and the Board of Certification cannot protect the copyright on the ATC mark if it becomes known as a common noun. Athletic trainers deliver rehabilitation services under a physician's guidelines.

Guidelines are general directions and descriptions that lead to the final outcome, thereby allowing the athletic trainer to rely on clinical decision making in constructing the rehabilitation protocol. Protocols are rigid step-by-step instructions that are common in technical fields and do not allow flexibility and/or clinical decision making. Athletic trainers function under a physician's direction. The terms *direction* and *supervision* mean 2 different things. Most importantly, supervision may require the on-site physical presence of the physician and that the physician examines each and every patient treated by an athletic trainer. Direction, however, requires contact and

Gorse KM, Feld F, Blanc RO, eds.
*Athletic Training Case Scenarios:
Domain-Based Situations and Solutions* (pp 243-244).
© 2016 Taylor & Francis Group.

interaction but not necessarily physical presence. Athletic trainers refer to the population that receives their services as patients or clients. Athletes comprise a significant proportion of the population who receive care from athletic trainers. However, once an athlete (or any other individual) becomes injured, he or she is a patient. The term *client* should be used for situations in which individuals receive athletic training services—usually preventive in nature—on a fee-for-service basis. Athletic trainers refer to secondary school and college-based work spaces as *facilities* or *clinics.* The term *athletic training room* does not appropriately recognize the health care services that are delivered within its walls. It may be impractical to find a one-term-fits-all descriptor to describe this area, and each institution/facility will use the most appropriate term for its venue. Athletic trainers should not use the term *board certified.* In medicine, the definition of *board certified* is a process to ensure that an individual has met standards beyond those of admission into licensure and has passed specialty examinations in the field. Various medical professional organizations establish their own board certification examinations. Although the term *board certified* is recognizable within the heath care and medical communities, based on the previous definition, the entry-level examination does not fit the criteria of being Board Certified. The recommended term is *certified athletic trainer.*

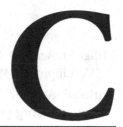

Suggested Readings in Athletic Training

American Academy of Orthopaedic Surgeons. *Emergency Care and Transportation of the Sick and Injured.* 10th ed. Sudbury, MA: Jones and Bartlett; 2013.

American College of Sports Medicine. *ACSM's Guidelines for Exercise Testing and Prescription.* 9th ed. Philadelphia, PA: Lippincott Williams & Wilkins; 2013.

Anderson MK, Hall SJ, Martin M. *Foundations of Athletic Training: Prevention, Assessment, and Management.* 5th ed. Philadelphia, PA: Lippincott Williams & Wilkins; 2012.

Biel AB. *Trail Guide to the Body.* 4th ed. Boulder, CO: Books of Discovery; 2010.

Cuppett M, Walsh K. *General Medical Conditions in the Athlete.* 2nd ed. St. Louis, MO: Elsevier/Mosby, Inc; 2011.

France RC. *Introduction to Sports Medicine and Athletic Training.* 2nd ed. Clifton Park, NY: Delmar Cengage Learning; 2010.

Gorse KM, Feld F, Blanc R, Radelet M. *Emergency Care in Athletic Training.* Philadelphia, PA: F.A. Davis Company; 2009.

Harrelson G, Gardner G, Winterstein AP. *Administrative Topics in Athletic Training: Concepts to Practice.* Thorofare, NJ: SLACK Incorporated; 2009.

Houglum PA. *Therapeutic Exercise for Musculoskeletal Injuries.* 3rd ed. Champaign, IL: Human Kinetics; 2010.

Houglum J, Harrelson G. *Principles of Pharmacology for Athletic Trainers.* Thorofare, NJ: SLACK Incorporated; 2010.

Kutz MR. *Leadership and Management in Athletic Training: An Integrated Approach.* Philadelphia, PA: Lippincott Williams & Wilkins; 2009.

Gorse KM, Feld F, Blanc RO, eds.
Athletic Training Case Scenarios:
Domain-Based Situations and Solutions (pp 245-246).
© 2016 Taylor & Francis Group.

Miller M, Berry D. *Emergency Response Management for Athletic Trainers*. Philadelphia, PA: Lippincott Williams & Wilkins; 2010.

National Athletic Trainers' Association. Position statements. *NATA website*. http://www.nata.org/position-statements. Accessed April 23, 2015.

Perrin DH. *Athletic Taping and Bracing*. 3rd ed. Champaign, IL: Human Kinetics; 2012.

Pfeiffer RP, Mangus BC, Trowbridge C. *Concepts of Athletic Training*. 6th ed. Sudbury, MA: Jones & Bartlett Learning; 2011.

Prentice WE. *Principles of Athletic Training: A Competency-Based Approach*. 15th ed. Boston, MA: McGraw Hill; 2013.

Prentice WE. *Rehabilitation Techniques for Sports Medicine and Athletic Training*. 5th ed. Boston, MA: McGraw Hill; 2010.

Ray R, Konin J. *Management Strategies in Athletic Training*. 4th ed. Champaign, IL: Human Kinetics; 2011.

Schulz S, Houglum P, Perrin D. *Examination of Musculoskeletal Injuries*. 3rd ed. Champaign, IL: Human Kinetics; 2009.

Starkey C. *Athletic Training and Sports Medicine: An Integrated Approach*. 5th ed. Sudbury, MA: Jones & Bartlett Publishers; 2012.

Starkey C, Brown SD. *Examination of Orthopedic and Athletic Injuries*. 3rd ed. Philadelphia, PA: F.A. Davis Company; 2009.

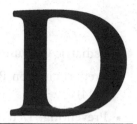

National Athletic Trainers' Association Position, Official, Consensus, and Support Statements

NATA POSITION STATEMENTS

http://www.nata.org/position-statements

- Acute Management of the Cervical Spine-Injured Athlete (2001)
- Anabolic-Androgenic Steroids (September 2012)
- Emergency Planning in Athletics (March 2002)
- Evaluation of Dietary Supplements for Performance Nutrition (February 2013)
- Exertional Heat Illnesses (September 2002)
- Fluid Replacement for Athletes (June 2000)
- Head-Down Contact and Spearing in Tackle Football (March 2004)
- Lightning Safety for Athletics and Recreation (March 2013)
- Management of Asthma in Athletes (September 2005)
- Management of Sport Concussion (March 2014)
- Management of Sport-Related Concussion (September 2004)
- Management of the Athlete with Type 1 Diabetes Mellitus (December 2007)
- National Athletic Trainers' Association Position Statement: Preventing Sudden Death in Sports (February 2012)
- National Athletic Trainers' Association Position Statement: Safe Weight Loss and Maintenance Practices in Sport and Exercise (June 2011)

Gorse KM, Feld F, Blanc RO, eds.
Athletic Training Case Scenarios:
Domain-Based Situations and Solutions (pp 247-249).
© 2016 Taylor & Francis Group.

- Pediatric Overuse Injuries (April 2011)

- Preparticipation Physical Examinations and Disqualifying Conditions (February 2014)

- Preventing, Detecting, and Managing Disordered Eating in Athletes (February 2008)

NATA OFFICIAL STATEMENTS

http://www.nata.org/official-statements
- Automated External Defibrillators (2003)

- Calling Crown of the Helmet Violations (August 2013)

- Commotio Cordis (October 2007)

- Communicable and Infectious Diseases in Secondary School Sports (March 2007)

- Community-Acquired MRSA Infections (March 2005)

- Full-Time, On-Site Athletic Trainer Coverage for Secondary School Athletic Programs

- Pre-Hospital Care of the Athlete with Cervical Spine Injury (May 2014)

- Proper Supervision of Secondary School Student Aides (June 2014)

- Providing Quality Health Care and Safeguards to Athletes of All Ages and Levels of Participation (December 2011)

- Steroids and Performance Enhancing Substances (March 2005)

- Use of Qualified Athletic Trainers in Secondary Schools (February 2004)

- Youth Football and Heat Related Illness (July 2005)

NATA CONSENSUS STATEMENTS

http://www.nata.org/consensus-statements
- Acute Management of the Cervical Spine Injured Athlete Position Statement

- Appropriate Medical Care for Secondary School-age Athletes (February 2003)

- Inter-Association Consensus Statement on Best Practices for Sports Medicine Management for Secondary Schools and Colleges

- Inter-Association Recommendations in Developing a Plan for Recognition and Referral of Student-Athletes with Psychological Concerns at the Collegiate Level

- Inter-Association Recommendations on Emergency Preparedness and Management of Sudden Cardiac Arrest in High School and College Athletic Programs (March 2007)

- Inter-Association Task Force for Preventing Sudden Death in Collegiate Conditioning Sessions: Best Practices Recommendations
- Inter-Association Task Force on Exertional Heat Illnesses (June 2003)
- Managing Prescriptions and Non-prescription Medication in the Athletic Training Facility (January 2009)
- Prehospital Care of the Spine-injured Athlete (2001)
- Preseason Heat-Acclimatization Guidelines for Secondary School Athletics (2009)
- Preventing Sudden Death in Secondary School Athletics
- Sickle Cell Trait and the Athlete

NATA SUPPORT STATEMENTS

http://www.nata.org/support-statements

- American Academy of Family Physicians' Support of Athletic Trainers for High School Athletes (2007)
- American Medical Association's Support of Athletic Trainers in Secondary Schools (July 1998)
- Appropriate Medical Care for Secondary School-age Athletes (Manuscript) (2004)
- Endorsement of NATA Lightning Position Statement by the American Academy of Pediatrics (April 2002)
- NCAA Support of Recommendations and Guidelines for Appropriate Medical Coverage of Intercollegiate Athletics (August 2003)
- Recommendations and Guidelines for Appropriate Medical Coverage of Intercollegiate Athletics
- The Coalition to Preserve Patient Access to Physical Medicine and Rehabilitation Services (December 2005)

Bibliography

American Heart Association. Guidelines 2010 for cardiopulmonary resuscitation and emergency cardiovascular care: international consensus on science. *Curr Emerg Cardiovasc Care*. 2010;11:3-15.

Anderson J, Courson RW, Kleiner DM, McLoda TA. National Athletic Trainers' Association Position Statement: emergency planning in athletics. *J Athl Train*. 2002;37(1):99-104.

Binkley HM, Beckett J, Casa DJ, Kleiner DM, Plummer PE. National Athletic Trainers' Association Position Statement: exertional heat illness. *J Athl Train*. 2002;37(3):329-343.

Board of Certification. *Role Delineation Study*. 6th ed. Raleigh, NC: Castle Worldwide; 2010.

Board of Certification, Continuing Education Office. *Continuing Education File 2006-2008*. Dallas, TX: Board of Certification; 2007.

Casa DJ, Armstrong LE, Hillmann SK, et al. National Athletic Trainers' Association Position Statement: fluid replacement for athletes. *J Athl Train*. 2000;35(2):212-224.

Federal Emergency Management Agency. National incident management system. http://www.fema.gov/national-incident-management-system. Updated April 21, 2015. Accessed April 23, 2015.

Guskiewicz KM, Bruce SL, Cantu RC, et al. National Athletic Trainers' Association Position Statement: management of sport-related concussion. *J Athl Train*. 2004;39(3):280-297.

National Athletic Trainers' Association. NATA website. www.nata.org. Accessed April 23, 2015.

Gorse KM, Feld F, Blanc RO, eds.
Athletic Training Case Scenarios:
Domain-Based Situations and Solutions (pp 251-252).
© 2016 Taylor & Francis Group.

National Athletic Trainers' Association. *2001 Standards and Guidelines*. Dallas, TX: National Athletic Trainers' Association; 2001.

National Athletic Trainers' Association. *NATA Code of Ethics*. Dallas, TX: National Athletic Trainers' Association; 2005.

National Athletic Trainers' Association. *Certification Update*. Dallas, TX: National Athletic Trainers' Association Board of Certification; 2000.

National Athletic Trainers' Association. *Athletic Training Educational Competencies*. 5th ed. Dallas, TX: National Athletic Trainers' Association Education Council; 2010.

National Collegiate Athletic Association. *2012-2013 Sports Medicine Handbook*. Indianapolis, IN: National Collegiate Athletic Association; 2012.

Financial Disclosures

Jon Almquist has not disclosed any relevant financial relationships.

Adam Annaccone has not disclosed any relevant financial relationships.

Robert O. Blanc has no financial or proprietary interest in the materials presented herein.

Lynn Bott has not disclosed any relevant financial relationships.

Rick Burr has not disclosed any relevant financial relationships.

Rex Call has no financial or proprietary interest in the materials presented herein.

Eric Cardwell has not disclosed any relevant financial relationships.

Dr. Douglas J. Casa has not disclosed any relevant financial relationships.

Robert J. Casmus has no financial or proprietary interest in the materials presented herein.

Craig Castor has not disclosed any relevant financial relationships.

Dr. Jim Cerullo has no financial or proprietary interest in the materials presented herein.

Dr. Kevin M. Conley has not disclosed any relevant financial relationships.

Larry Cooper has not disclosed any relevant financial relationships.

Ron Courson has no financial or proprietary interest in the materials presented herein.

Dr. Jennifer Doherty-Restrepo has no financial or proprietary interest in the materials presented herein.

A. J. Duffy III has no financial or proprietary interest in the materials presented herein.

Tim Dunlavey has not disclosed any relevant financial relationships.

Francis Feld has no financial or proprietary interest in the materials presented herein.

Scott Frowen has not disclosed any relevant financial relationships.

Timothy K. Giel has not disclosed any relevant financial relationships.

Dr. Keith M. Gorse has no financial or proprietary interest in the materials presented herein.

Al Green has no financial or proprietary interest in the materials presented herein.

Michael Hanley has not disclosed any relevant financial relationships.

Kelley Henderson has no financial or proprietary interest in the materials presented herein.

Dr. Timothy J. Henry has not disclosed any relevant financial relationships.

Dr. Valerie W. Herzog has no financial or proprietary interest in the materials presented herein.

Adam M. Hindes has not disclosed any relevant financial relationships.

Peter Houdek has not disclosed any relevant financial relationships.

Dr. Peggy A. Houglum has not disclosed any relevant financial relationships.

Chuck Kimmel has no financial or proprietary interest in the materials presented herein.

Mary K. Kirkland has not disclosed any relevant financial relationships.

Catherine S. Lenhardt has not disclosed any relevant financial relationships.

Dr. Sarah Manspeaker has not disclosed any relevant financial relationships.

Christopher Marrone has not disclosed any relevant financial relationships.

Randy McGuire has not disclosed any relevant financial relationships.

Jennifer McKenzie has not disclosed any relevant financial relationships.

Dr. Linda P. Meyer has no financial or proprietary interest in the materials presented herein.

Dr. Sayers John Miller has not disclosed any relevant financial relationships.

Mary Mundrane-Zweiacher has not disclosed any relevant financial relationships.

Kathleen Nachazel has not disclosed any relevant financial relationships.

Gregory Nordlund has no financial or proprietary interest in the materials presented herein.

John Panos has not disclosed any relevant financial relationships.

Dr. David H. Perrin has not disclosed any relevant financial relationships.

Ben Potenziano has not disclosed any relevant financial relationships.

Marirose Radelet has not disclosed any relevant financial relationships.

Matthew Radelet has not disclosed any relevant financial relationships.

Jeramiah Randall has no financial or proprietary interest in the materials presented herein.

Dr. Richard Ray has not disclosed any relevant financial relationships.

Joan Reed has not disclosed any relevant financial relationships.

Christopher Rose has not disclosed any relevant financial relationships.

Gaetano Sanchioli has not disclosed any relevant financial relationships.

Dr. Bonnie J. Siple has no financial or proprietary interest in the materials presented herein.

Dr. Rebecca L. Stearns has not disclosed any relevant financial relationships.

Charles Thompson has no financial or proprietary interest in the materials presented herein.

Todd Tomczyk has not disclosed any relevant financial relationships.

Dr. Paula S. Turocy has not disclosed any relevant financial relationships.

Dr. Giampietro L. Vairo has no financial or proprietary interest in the materials presented herein.

Brian Vesci has not disclosed any relevant financial relationships.

Michael Vittorino has not disclosed any relevant financial relationships.

Mary C. Wisniewski has no financial or proprietary interest in the materials presented herein.

Index

abdominal injuries
in football, 115-116
in soccer, 105-106
accreditation violation, in baseball, 207-208
Achilles tendon injuries
in football, 159-160
in spectators, 109-110
airway management, in head injuries, 139-140
amplified muscle pain syndrome, in running, 63-64
ankle range of motion deficiency, in squatting exercise, 151-152
ankle sprains
in ballet dancing, 45-46
in baseball, 157-158
in basketball, 17-18
in softball, 145-146
arm. *See also* elbow injuries; shoulder injuries
lacerations of
after basketball practice, 131-132
in football, 95-96

arteriovenous malformation, of brain, 31-34
asthma
in soccer, 5-6
in swimming, 211-212
ATC acronym, 243-244
Athletic Training Program
closure of, 205-206
justifying during tough financial times, 187-188
athletic training room, 244

back pain
in baseball, 55-56
in rowing, 169-170
in track and field sports, 223-224
ballet dancing, ankle sprains in, 45-46
baseball and softball
ankle sprains in, 145-146
collision injuries in, 55-56
concussion in, 57-58
facial injuries in, 49-50, 193-194
knee injuries in, 183-184
lower leg injuries in, 133-134

os trigonum fractures in, 157-158

outreach athletic trainer services in, 197-198

overuse injuries in, 155-156

shoulder injuries and pain in, 51-54, 161-162

Spanish-speaking athletes in, 221-222

subscapular bursitis in, 161-162

trainer accreditation violation in, 207-208

trainer communication problems in, 217-219

basketball

ankle sprains in, 17-18

arm injury after practice, 131-132

cervical spinal injuries in, 135-136

biceps, myositis ossificans in, in football, 153-154

board certification, of athletic trainers, 244

bomb threat, during running events, 173-174

brain. *See also* concussion

arteriovenous malformation in, 31-34

subdural hematoma of, 101-102

breathing dysfunction, in football, 43-44

bursitis, subscapular, in baseball catcher, 161-162

Business Associates Agreement, 201-202

cardiovascular disease, chest pain in, 123-124

certification, of athletic trainers, 244

cervical spine injuries

in basketball, 135-136

in diving, 99-100

in football, 87, 117-118, 175-176, 189-191

challenges, among personnel. *See* conflict

cheerleading, stress fractures in, 13-14

chest pain, in cardiovascular disease, 123-124

chiropractic care, 223-224

clinical evaluation, 31-88

coaching staff, disagreement with

in soccer, 9-10

in softball, 183-184

collision injuries

in baseball, 55-56

in soccer, 111-112, 195-196

communication

during bomb threat, in running events, 173-174

with language barriers, 221-222

problems with

in athletic department, 217-219

in cervical spine injuries, 135-136

concussion

in baseball, 57-58

in football, 59-60, 69-70, 147-148

in soccer, 9-10

confidentiality, social media and, 185-186

conflict

with coaching staff

in soccer, 9-10

in softball, 183-184

with college administration, over athletic training program, 205-206

with emergency care personnel

in football helmet removal, 189-191

in soccer, 195-196

with health personnel, in soccer, 61-62

cooperation

with coaching personnel, 183-184

with emergency medical services, 175-176

lack of. *See* conflict

crew team. *See* rowing

cumulative trauma disorder, in information technology work, 167-168

deep vein thrombosis, after ankle sprains, 145-146

diagnosis, 31-88

direct supervision policy, violation of, 207-208

direction, in athletic training, 243-244

disagreement. *See* conflict

diversity, in athletic training, 213-214

diving, spinal injuries in, 99-100

drug use, in rowing, 179-180

eating disorders, in running, 149-150

elbow injuries

    in baseball, 155-156

    in football, 171-172

emergency care, 89-140, 171-172, 175-176

    conflict with

        in football helmet removal, 189-191

        in majorette injury, 215-216

        in soccer injury, 195-196

Ethnic Diversity Committee, of NATA, 213-214

facial fractures

    in pole vaulting, 107-108

    in soccer, 65-66, 91-92

facial injuries, in baseball and softball, 49-50, 193-194

fatigue, in running, 149-150

femoral fractures

    in football, 47-48

    in lacrosse, 35-36

fibular fractures, in football, 101-101

foot

    injuries of

        in football, 71-72

        in majorette, 215-216

    Staphylococcus infections of, 83-84

football

    abdominal injuries in, 115-116

    Achilles tendon reconstruction and, 159-160

    arm lacerations in, 95-96

    breathing dysfunction in, 43-44

    cervical spine injuries in, 87, 117-118, 175-176, 189-191

    concussion in, 19-20, 59-60, 69-70, 147-148

    elbow injuries in, 171-172

    emergency utilization in, 171-172

    femoral fractures in, 47-48

    fibular fractures in, 101-101

    foot fractures in, 71-72

    gunshots heard during, 7-8

    head injuries in, 31-34, 101-102, 129-130

    helmet removal in, 189-191

    hip injuries in, 125-128

    hyperthyroidism and, 39-40

    knee injuries in, 93-94, 109-110, 113-114, 141-143

    multiple injuries in, 109-110

    myocardial infarction in, 121-122

    myositis ossificans development and, 153-154

    rib injuries in, 41-42, 77-78

    shoulder pain in, 163-165

    social media comments about, 185-186

    squatting exercises in, 151-152

    Staphylococcus infections in, 83-84

    subdural hematoma in, 101-102

    thumb injury in, 37-38

    trainer unprofessional behavior in, 209-210

    wrist injuries in, 171-172

footwear

    ankle sprains due to, 17-18

    sensation of broken sole in, 71-72

fractures

    facial, in soccer, 65-66

    femoral

        in football, 47-48

        in running, 75-76

    fibular, in football, 101-101

    Lisfranc, in football, 71-72

    os trigonum, in baseball, 157-158

    rib, in football, 41-42

    stress. *See* stress fractures

golf, multiple sclerosis in, 85-86
Good Samaritan Law, 193-194
Graves' disease, football and, 39-40
gunshots, heard during football practice,
    7-8

head injuries. *See also* concussion
    in football, 101-102, 129-130
    in pole vaulting, 107-108
    in soccer, 9-10, 91-92, 111-112
    in track, 139-140
    in wrestling, 89-90
health information, protected, 201-202
heat illness
    in lacrosse, 29-30
    in running, 73-74, 137-138
    in spectators, 97-98
helicopter transport, for head injuries,
    129-130
hematoma, subdural, in football, 101-102
herpes gladiatorum, in wrestling, 15-16,
    25-26
hip injuries
    in football, 125-128
    in weight room, 67-68
hockey, shoulder injuries in, 23-24
Homeland Security, contacting during
    running events, 173-174
hydromyelia, in running, 63-64
hyperthyroidism, football and, 39-40

ice hockey, shoulder injuries in, 23-24
illness prevention, 3-30
immediate care. *See* emergency care
impetigo, in wrestling, 15-16
incident command system, for terrorist
    threats, 173-174
information technology work, cumulative
    trauma disorder in, 167-168
inhaler, for asthma, 5-6
injuries. *See also specific locations*
    prevention of, 3-30

insurance coverage, in emergency utiliza-
    tion, 171-172
interphalangeal joint, of thumb, injury of,
    37-38
interpreters, for foreign language speak-
    ers, 221-222
iron supplementation, for fatigue, in run-
    ning, 149-150

jet skiing, liver laceration in, 115-116

knee injuries
    in baseball, 55-56
    in football, 93-94, 109-110, 113-114,
        141-143
    physician referral for, 203-204
    in running, 63-64
    in soccer, 61-62, 79-80, 91-92
    in softball, 183-184

lacrosse
    heat illness in, 29-30
    shin protection in, 3-4
    splenic injuries in, 119-120
    stress fractures in, 35-36, 181-182
language barriers, 135-136, 221-222
licensing, problems with, 193-194
Lisfranc fractures, in football, 71-72
liver lacerations, in jet skiing, 115-116

magnetic resonance imaging, long wait-
    ing times for, 67-68
majorette, foot injury in, 215-216
mallet injuries, of thumb, in football, 37-38
medical chain of authority, for return to
    play, 211-212
medications, dispensed by athletic trainer,
    27-28
minority population, representation in
    athletic training, 213-214
multiple injuries
    in football, 109-110
    in soccer, 91-92

multiple sclerosis, in golf, 85-86

myocardial infarction, in football, 121-122

myositis ossificans development, in football, 153-154

National Athletic Trainers' Association
consensus statements of, 248-249
mission of, 243
official statements of, 248
position statements of, 247-248
support statements of, 249
terminology of, 243-244
National Incident Management System, 173-174

orbital fractures, in soccer, 65-66

organizational issues, for athletic trainers, 171-224

os trigonum fractures, in baseball, 157-158

osteopenia, stress fractures in, 13-14

overuse injuries, in baseball, 155-156

parental conflict, in knee injury rehabilitation, 141-143

patellar tendon ruptures, in football, 113-114

Performance Team, wellness programs developed by, 11-12

personality alterations, in concussion, 59-60

physician, conflict with emergency medical services, 203-204

physician assistant, responsibility of, 217-219

pole vaulting, head injuries in, 107-108

policy and procedure
circumvention of, in back pain, 223-224
manuals for, 199-200

posttraumatic stress disorder, in concussion, 147-148

preceptors, accreditation violation by, 207-208

private information, on social media, 185-186

procedure manuals, 199-200

professional behavior, 209-210

professional health considerations, for athletic trainers, 171-224

protected health information, 201-202

psychological issues, in concussion, 147-148

public safety, in running events, 173-174

races. *See* running

referral, to physician, 203-204

rehabilitation, 141-170

response time, of emergency services, 95-96

return to play, in swimming, 211-212

rib fractures and injuries, in football, 41-42, 77-78

rowing
athlete drug use in, 179-180
back pain in, 169-170

running
amplified muscle pain syndrome in, 63-64
bomb threat during, 173-174
fatigue in, 149-150
femoral fractures in, 75-76
heat illness in, 73-74, 137-138

shin protection, in lacrosse, 3-4

shoes. *See* footwear

shoulder injuries
in baseball, 51-54, 161-162
in football, 41-42, 163-165
in hockey, 23-24
in rowing, 169-170

small intestinal injuries, in soccer, 105-106

soccer
abdominal trauma in, 105-106
asthma in, 5-6
coach disagreement during, 9-10

collision injuries in, 111-112, 195-196

facial fractures in, 65-66

head injuries in, 9-10, 91-92, 111-112

health personnel disagreement in, 61-62

knee injuries in, 79-80, 91-92

multiple injured persons in, 91-92

social media, football team information on, 185-186

softball. *See* baseball and softball

spectators

heat illness in, 97-98

leg injuries in, 109-110

spinal injuries

cervical. *See* cervical spine injuries

in diving, 99-100

in football, 87, 117-118

in track sports, 223-224

splenic injuries

in baseball, 55-56

in lacrosse, 119-120

sports medicine team, emergency utilization of, in football, 171-172

sprains, ankle. *See* ankle sprains

squatting exercises, in football, 151-152

Staphylococcus infections, in football, 83-84

stress fractures

in cheerleading, 13-14

in lacrosse, 35-36, 181-182

in running, 75-76

in track sports, 223-224

subclavian vein thrombosis, in volleyball, 81-82

subdural hematoma, in football, 101-102

subscapular bursitis, in baseball catcher, 161-162

supervision, in athletic training, 243-244

swelling, after ankle sprains, 145-146

swimming

asthma in, return to play after, 211-212

spinal injuries in, 99-100

terminology, of athletic training, 243-244

thrombosis, upper extremity, in volleyball, 81-82

throwing sports

overuse injuries in, 155-156

shoulder pain in, 51-54, 161-162, 163-165

thumb, mallet injury of, in football, 37-38

tibiotalar dislocation, in wrestling, 177-178

track and field. *See also* running

back pain in, policy circumvention in, 223-224

head injuries in, 107-108, 139-140

stress fractures in, 13-14

translators, for foreign language speakers, 221-222

travel outside university area, trainer responsibility in, 217-219

treatment and rehabilitation, 141-170

triage, 91-92

ulnar collateral ligament repair, after throwing injuries, 155-156

unprofessional behavior, 209-210

upper extremity effort thrombosis, in volleyball, 81-82

vertebrae, stress fractures of, in track sports, 223-224

vocal cord dysfunction, paradoxical, in football, 43-44

volleyball

eating disorders and, 21-22

upper extremity effort thrombosis in, 81-82

weight room, hip injuries in, 67-68

wellness program, development of, 11-12

wellness protection, 3-30

work station, cumulative trauma disorder at, 167-168

wrestling
    head injuries in, 89-90
    skin conditions in, 15-16, 25-26
    tibiotalar dislocation in, 177-178
wrist injuries, in football, 171-172

zygomatic bone fractures
    in soccer, 65-66
    in softball, 49-50

Printed in the United States
by Baker & Taylor Publisher Services